# Sexuality and

TRUST

LIBRARY

## A guide for everyday practice

## ELAINE COOPER

*Consultant Advisor on Sexuality Issues*
*Southampton Community Health Services NHS Trust*

and

## JOHN GUILLEBAUD

*Medical Director*
*Margaret Pyke Family Planning Centre*

Foreword by

## MORGAN WILLIAMS

RADCLIFFE MEDICA

Radcliffe Medical Press Ltd
18 Marcham Road, Abingdon, Oxon OX14 1AA

British Library Cataloguing in Publication Data

A catalogue record for this book is available from the British Library.

ISBN 1 85775 319 4

Typeset by Action Publishing Technology, Gloucester
Printed and bound by Biddles Ltd, Guildford and King's Lynn

# Contents

# Foreword

The poet Philip Larkin may have discovered sex in 1963 but for people with a disability the discovery came several years later. Or, more accurately, the realisation by professional carers that disabled people have similar emotional, sexual and relationship needs as their more able-bodied peers.

In the early 1970s, the late Dr Duncan Guthrie recruited some like-minded friends and colleagues to form the Committee on Sexual Problems of the Disabled (SPOD). The name has changed and evolved over the years to reflect awareness and political correctness, but for all that it is still generally known as SPOD.

The original committee did an enormous amount to raise awareness in the disability sector through contacts in disability organisations and its promotion in 1979 of the first ever International Conference on Sexuality and Disability. In the late 1970s the committee also supported a research project, conducted by the late Bill Stewart, that is still considered the research benchmark on sexuality and disability. Initially, this discovery led to a proliferation of publications, particularly by Ann and Michael Craft and Wendy Greengross. However, by the late 1980s (with the exception of one or two books by the late Ann Craft) all were out of print with no plans for future editions.

Somehow the assumption was that having identified the sexual needs of disabled people – I hesitate to use the word 'problems' – all had been resolved. Far from it. In 15 years as Director of SPOD, that latterly included facilitating workshops, I realised that the problems were usually with the carers and not the client group. The vast majority of disabled people were aware of what they could and could not do, whom they wanted to do it with, when and where. The problems mostly began for them when they needed to ask a carer for help, e.g. buying contraceptives, taking them to a social event, making an appointment, lifting them into bed with a partner or just affording them privacy. That often seemed to be the signal for the carer to project their own value system on to the situation and frequently say 'No', using risk as the reason.

So, I heartily welcome this book and commend it to you. Elaine Cooper and John Guillebaud have compiled a unique and valuable resource that not only covers every disability but presents everything in such a matter of fact and reasonable way. My only regret is that there is no ruling that would make these excellent strategies enforceable. I wonder how often carers consider how they would like it to be for themselves if they were to acquire a disability, and realise that sexuality and relationships are part of the whole person whether or not they have a disability.

Morgan Williams
Former Director of SPOD
*May 1999*

# Preface

When I began to work with people with disabilities in the domiciliary family planning service, two main facts struck me. First, very few people with disabilities attended family planning clinics and I was initially seeing small numbers on my visits. Liaising with the general practitioners, they seemed to see even fewer people. Were people with disability accessing services or were they being neglected? Secondly, the unease expressed by health professionals and others when sexuality and disability was raised. Many have said to me over the years 'you should write something about this, it would be so helpful'. Here is the result, and I hope that it will be helpful and valuable in improving the service provided for people with disabilities.

Elaine Cooper
*May 1999*

# Acknowledgements

When I first decided to write I was encouraged by Ruth Skrine, Jeanette Cayley, Morgan Williams and John Guillebaud, all of whose opinion I asked about the idea of this book. John Guillebaud was so supportive he offered to be my co-author. I am grateful also to my colleague Professor Lindsay McLellan for reading the text and his valuable comments, and to Morgan Williams for writing the foreword.

My gratitude to the staff of Radcliffe Medical Press, Heidi, Gregory, Jamie and Paula, for their guidance. A very big thank you to my secretary Isabel Wright for her patience and commitment in typing the text.

I particularly want to acknowledge the continuing encouragement and support given by my children, Alison, Jonathan and Geoffrey, not only at this time but throughout the years. A special thank you to Jonathan and his wife Alison for reading the first draft and making comments and offering advice. My husband David has been a constant presence and supporter of my work for nearly forty years. He has lived with this book and spent many hours revising the text with me. I cannot thank him enough.

Finally, thank you to my colleagues of all disciplines and most especially those people with disabilities with whom I have worked and who have taught me so much about living with disability.

Elaine Cooper
*May 1999*

# Author note

In the interest of anonymity no real names are used, they are all allocated in alphabetical order. If any reader believes they can recognise themselves in the case studies it is likely that they are identifying with someone else with a similar story. They can be assured that no one else will recognise them. Throughout the text, except in matters of fertility, what is said would generally apply to either heterosexual or homosexual activity.

... In a society in which there is genuine respect for the handi-
capped; where understanding is unostentatious and sincere;
where if years cannot be added to the lives of the very sick, at least
life can be added to their years ...

Alf Morris MP in presenting the Bill for the Chronically Sick
and Disabled Persons Act for the second reading

# CHAPTER 1

# Counselling and sexuality

When counselling any person, disabled or not, about issues relating to sexuality it is important to ensure that the work is patient-centred and it is carried out with sensitivity, because these are very personal and private areas of a person's life. It is an area where individual choice is paramount. It is essential that the views of the professional are not allowed to intrude upon the consultation and that it is non-judgemental.

People need to be assured that confidentiality will be upheld at all times and that except where the personal safety of another individual is at risk (e.g. abuse), information will not be revealed. Alongside this, of course, it is important that privacy is available, both visual and auditory.

Where people with disabilities are being counselled there are other areas of concern to consider. The most obvious of these is accessibility. In the 1990s new buildings are required to have disabled access but in some older buildings this is not possible. In these circumstances it may be that there is a need to take the service to the person (e.g. by visiting at their home, day centre or training centre). It is important to have a venue where privacy is guaranteed and uninterrupted by other family members or staff. Counselling on a ward with only curtain screening is inappropriate as although visually screened, the consultation can be overheard by other people on the ward.

# Physical disability

Comprehension for people with physical disabilities is not a problem unless there is impairment of understanding, which may be due to head injury, stroke or more advanced stages of some neurological diseases. It is, of course, essential to communicate in a clear way using normal vocabulary and not medicalised jargon. Where vision or hearing is impaired it is important to be aware of this so as to assure that communication is good (e.g. when a general practitioner drew pictures about a method of contraception for a blind woman it was not helpful! Both the woman and the doctor became exasperated at their lack of communication and understanding). It is important to ascertain from the client how they are best able to communicate (e.g. if lip-reading is essential ensuring that the counsellor's face is in a good light and turned towards the client).

Some people are aphasic and communicate by other means such as Makaton signing or using a Bliss board* or a computer. It is for the counsellor to take a lead from the client who will be experienced in their chosen mode of communication.

# Learning disability

When working with people with learning disability, ascertaining that they have fully understood what is being said is essential. They may not have the words to communicate their feelings and needs. Enquiry as to their words (e.g. for parts of the body) is important so that real contact can occur. In addition, some people need time to assimilate a question and it is important to allow them to formulate an answer before another question is asked. It is important to work at their pace and to ask single questions rather than complicated questions with choices. For example, for some people asking, 'do you mean $x$ or $y$?' can be too complicated, whereas to be asked about $x$ and a reply given before $y$ is raised provides real answers. The usual style of open-ended questions

*Makaton: a form of sign language. *Bliss board*: a board containing squares in each of which is a symbol, letter or phrase used to aid communication.

may be too difficult and counselling styles may need to be adapted. Unless these adaptations are made the response may be incorrect or 'I don't know' or sometimes a completely unrelated response may occur like 'I am going out to tea today'. These responses may mean 'I don't know', or may be an escape route to closing a difficult or painful topic.

Sometimes, carers, professional or family, may wish to be involved in the consultation. It is important to ascertain that the client is in agreement with this. The client may ask for the carer to be present as this increases the client's confidence. Carers undoubtedly have concerns and anxieties, not least their responsibility to the client, and this can sometimes mean that the carer may take on a high profile in the consultation and speak for the client, even when they can communicate for themselves! It may be very important to involve the carer, especially where assistance in implementing actions explored in the consultation may be necessary (e.g. changes in behavioural patterns). This is particularly so where there is only short-term memory and the consultation quickly forgotten.

Where there is severe or profound learning disability, issues about consent need to be investigated – most especially informed consent. An assessment of competence is necessary. It is essential to work within an ethical and legal framework, in the person's best interest.

Of course, as in the non-disabled population, there will be some people who will have anxieties about their sexual orientation. Because of some attitudes to same-sex relationships, exploring these anxieties can be inhibited by fear of prejudgement by the professional. Where there are fears about attitudes to disability it compounds the difficulty. People with learning disability may lack the words or other skills to access help. Those working with such people need to be aware of this. In general psychosexual services it appears that consultations concerning gender are increasing. These issues arise for people with disabilities too and there is a tendency for them to be brushed aside and not to be addressed. This does the individuals a disservice: it is often quite difficult for people with learning disabilities to have their questions taken seriously.

# CHAPTER 2

# Society: the climate in which we live

There is a tendency for the 'the disabled' to be lumped together as one homogeneous entity, whereas, of course, each person with a disability is unique in both their personality and disability. There may be similarities to others with the same diagnosis, but above all each person should be considered as an individual. Many people who have disabilities are discriminated against or feel discriminated against in most areas of their lives, not least concerning their sexuality. 'I did not think people who are disabled would be interested in that sort of thing' or 'Disabled people don't do that (have sex) and if they do, they shouldn't'. This is sometimes summed up as 'society's attitude' as if society is an entity itself. We need to remember that we are all part of society, so must bear some responsibility for this attitude. Disabled people and their partners are also part of society and not separate beings. Where a disabling illness or accident occurs, these preconceived thoughts and feelings can damage or inhibit a sexual relationship. 'Sex is for the young, beautiful and athletic' seems to be the media message. If you are young, beautiful and athletic, then it is fine, but it leaves out many people including vast numbers of the general population, the so-called 'normal' population, many of whom do not fit the image and experience discomfort about their appearance or body image, by being too fat, too thin, too short, too tall, and so on.

For people with a visible disability the defined media image is distorted, as it is too for people with learning disability who may have a different facies and behave in a manner that does not fit the stereotyped image. Elderly people can be sidelined since after a 'certain age', sexual activity is not expected to occur. This age tends to increase as the age of the 'observer' increases! People who are wheelchair users often say that people only see the 'chair', they do not see the person in the chair. They become the disability plus John or Mary, rather than John or Mary who happens to be disabled and has the same anxieties, pleasures and needs as everyone else with perhaps some extra difficulties in addition.

Confronted with someone with a disability some people will endeavour to ignore the disability altogether. This is difficult for the disabled person as their disability is an integral part of them and need not, and should not, be ignored. Because we are all part of society, these attitudes affect partners, potential partners, parents and other carers and the professional and thus, as a consequence, the person with the disability.

**Case study A**

Anne, a young woman who had been blind since she was 3 years old, expressed great relief that she had a home visit from the family planning doctor. She felt unable to attend a clinic as she felt everyone would stare at her (although she could not see them) and be thinking or saying, 'what is she doing here in a family planning clinic, surely she has no sexual relationship, she is blind'.

**Case study B**

Bronwen stopped attending the clinic to have her IUD (intrauterine device) checked. On being contacted by the receptionist she confessed to feeling embarrassed at having to attend since her second leg had been amputated. She felt her gait was more obvious now she had two artificial legs. 'Everyone watches me walk across the waiting room and wonders how I come to be there when I am disabled.' She felt uncomfortable being clumsy when needing to get on to the couch for examination, especially if she felt the need to remove her artificial limbs.

Where there is a congenital disability or a disability has arisen in childhood there is a tendency to be protective and to see the person as being suspended in childhood (see Chapter 7). Where a child has a learning disability this attitude is more pronounced. The skills individuals with a learning disability have are variable. They may be five years old with respect to understanding and feeding themselves, but show other levels in their speech and other life skills. But adolescence occurs, and the concomitant hormonal changes will produce body and emotional changes as in all young people (see Chapter 7). However, there are some myths around sexuality and learning disability. These vary from 'no sense and so no feeling' to 'at it all the time' and 'will breed like rabbits'. Another widely held view is that 'if you do not tell them about sex they won't do it'. Any of these misapprehensions leave the person very vulnerable.

Talking to parents of people with learning disability, they are concerned that their children will be exploited by others and taken advantage of. This may be in the form of abuse (see below). They are anxious that their daughters will become pregnant and that either sex will contract infection, especially HIV and AIDS. To deal with this there is a 'lock up your daughters' response from some in an endeavour to keep them safe. This then denies the person the opportunity to form relationships and broaden their experience of life. An alternative to this limiting way of dealing with the situation is to give the person information and guidance to prepare them and so reduce the risks of exploitation and abuse, unplanned pregnancy and infection.

When working with people with learning disabilities, during a consultation it is frequently found that there is a great deal of ignorance or misunderstanding in their sexual knowledge concerning the body's function and behaviour. It is often apparent that there has been little sex education or perhaps it was inappropriately delivered. For example, it may have been given to a group where it is difficult to meet individual needs. In those circumstances it may not have appeared relevant to them. There is often a need for sex education in the consultation which is done on a one-to-one basis. There are obviously many restrictions in providing one-to-one education for everyone in schools or colleges because of constraints on time, staff and finance resources. It is possible, of course, that information has been given and forgotten, especially if it did not seem relevant. It is clear that for many older people with learning disabilities provision of sex education would have either not been considered or it would have been deemed irrelevant, as it was perceived they would be unlikely to have sexual relationships. It has been noted by staff working with physically disabled pupils in mainstream schools that the latter seem to feel that the sex education given to the non-disabled pupils is irrelevant to them.

The impression is often given to people with learning disability that they are 'being naughty' if they try to indulge in sexual relationships or activity, and although this feeling of naughtiness can add a frisson of excitement, it often brings feelings of guilt and the need to hide. This situation can be all the more difficult when the person may not have the language ability to express what they feel.

Not infrequently, the client will hasten to say in a consultation that 'it's not dirty' as if to dispel that suggestion and to be reassured. There can be very conflicting feelings when the desire for a relationship exists, and fear that there will be punishment for this behaviour. It would appear that, in some cases, those in responsibility (parent or professional carer) are understandably anxious to maintain the well-being of the person with the disability, to protect them from consequences and the need to avoid potentially risky behaviour and relationships. This anxiety in the parent/carer is often perceived as disapproval by the person with the disability, which makes it difficult for them to ask for help or guidance for fear of being 'told off'.

Another factor that increases the client's vulnerability is the tendency for people with disabilities to be told to behave themselves, to keep 'quiet' and to do as they are told. This engenders a feeling of 'must comply with instructions' and lays the person open to exploitation or abuse.

---

**Case study C**

Carol, a young woman with mild learning disability, reported that she had been raped by a person in responsibility who insisted on having sex with her. She did not want this to occur but felt unable to say no. She also explained she felt unable to make a sound and call for help, not because she was 'frozen' and lost her ability to speak, as is common in this situation, but because she was afraid that she would be told off for making a 'noise'. It would seem this young woman had been given information that was unhelpful in an emergency.

Closely related to this attitude is the issue of consent, which must be **informed** consent. When people have a disability and need medical or nursing intervention and intimate body care, it becomes 'routine' to be touched by others. Consent to such treatment should have been sought and given, but there comes a point when consent is implicit and compliance accepted. This means that in some ways the disabled person's body feels like 'public property'. They need to be assured that they are autonomous and they do not have to consent to anyone doing anything to them. In other words, it is within the person's right to say 'no'. They do not have to go along with any sexual approach made to them, the criterion being 'do I want/like this person to touch me in that way?'. Personal space is important and should not be invaded. People may need help to say 'no' or express 'no' if verbal communication is not possible.

The area of consent is very important in order to avoid abuse or exploitation but it is also of significance to the partner. Although people with physical disabilities, for the most part, have able minds and are able to make decisions like everyone else, the greatest problem may occur with learning disability. There may be anxieties if the relationship is between a woman with learning disability and a non-disabled man. In this situation, the man is also in a very vulnerable position, as he could readily be perceived as an abuser. It is essential that the relationship is open and not hidden, and that the woman is consenting. Indeed, not infrequently she may be the instigator of sexual activity. Openness about the relationship to parents or carers helps to safeguard against misunderstandings, and misjudgements of situations and allegations of misconduct.

It can be particularly difficult if an attraction develops between a non-disabled person who is a carer, man or woman, and a client of either sex. There may be a desire for a mutually happy, consensual relationship. Sexual relationships between carers and clients are not acceptable and are indeed grounds for dismissal. In this situation if their relationship was to continue and develop, it will be necessary for the carer to leave the care home and work elsewhere.

Although acknowledging that there may be difficulties for people with disabilities, it must never be assumed that there are always problems, any more than it should be thought that all non-disabled people have excellent relationships! Many people with disabilities have happy, fulfilling relationships and it would be presumptive and patronising to think otherwise. It is for the professional to have an awareness that there is a potential for sexual activity and hence also for sexual difficulty. In addition, there must be an awareness when working in the area of sexuality that cultural backgrounds and practices will vary and these need to be taken into consideration.

Many professionals working with people with disabilities (e.g. occupational therapists and physiotherapists) are uncertain how or when to broach the subject of sexuality. One way to deal with this is to build sensitive questions about sexual relationships into any assessment. Enquiry is often made concerning bowel or bladder function, or mobility. Including sexuality in this makes it part of normal life and not a separate entity. It is essential, of course, to have privacy when asking delicate questions. Art therapists are well placed to identify problems with sexuality especially in those people with limited communication. They are able to observe progress made as a result of counselling input.

## Abuse

Unfortunately, in our society sexual abuse exists and affects people of both sexes, of all ages, and the disabled and non-disabled. This may be isolated incidents, ongoing or within a continuing relationship. Coping with this is difficult for everyone, but there may be particular difficulties for someone with a disability both physically, because of frailty, and emotionally (see Chapter 3).

Even though there may be knowledge that agencies exist to

help, accessing them can be a problem due to lack of confidence and self-esteem, which is so common with both disability and abuse. Communication skills may be poor due to impairment. Some people will continue within the relationship in fear of their partner, being alone, being unable to cope, and not finding another partner, so may not wish to seek or accept assistance.

## Further reading

Brown H and Craft A (eds) (1989) *Thinking the Unthinkable*. FPA Education Unit, London.

Cooper E (1995) The needs of people with disability. *British Journal of Family Planning*. **21**(1): 31–2.

Craft A (ed) (1994) *Practice Issues in Sexuality and Learning Disabilities*. Routledge, London.

Fairbairn G *et al*. (1995) *Sexuality, Learning Difficulties and Doing What's Right*. David Fulton, London.

Gunn MJ (1996) *Sex and The Law: a brief guide for staff working with people with learning disabilities*. Family Planning Association, London.

Holmes J (1995) *Sexuality and Disability: the way forward*. Report on a conference held on 15 February 1995. Contact a Family, London.

McCarthy M and Cambridge P (1996) *Your Rights About Sex: a booklet for people with learning disabilities*. BILD Publications, Plymouth.

Owen OG (1994) Sex, contraception and disability. *British Journal of Sexual Medicine*. **21**(5): S1–S4.

Patterson-Keels L *et al*. (1994) Family views on sterilization for their mentally retarded children. *Journal of Reproductive Medicine*. **39**(9): 701–6.

Shakespeare T *et al*. (1996) *The Sexual Politics of Disability*. Cassell, London.

Shevlin M and McCormick G (1997) *Exploring Sexuality and Disability: walk your talk*. Family Planning Association, London.

Taylor G. *et al*. (1998) Family planning for women with learning disabilities. *Nursing Times*. **94**(40): 60–1.

# CHAPTER **3**

# Emotional factors

For anything that happens to us there is an emotional response, whether it is something we do or something that is beyond our control, because we all have feelings about these happenings. This applies also to those being born with or acquiring a disability. Emotional response will vary both by feelings experienced by the person with the disability themselves, about themselves and by the attitudes and emotional responses of other people around them to the disability.

Some people with an acquired disability may have had strong negative feelings about disabled people prior to their own accident or illness and this will affect how they feel about themselves, to be suddenly part of this 'labelled' group. They may, of course, believe that other people, partners or potential partners, may view them in a similar negative way. The difficulties highlighted in Chapter 2 will apply. It is important to understand what the disability means to each individual. The loss of function in an arm or a leg, the fact that it 'malfunctions' and may be held in a particular position (e.g. spastic contractures) may mean more to the individual than a practical problem. It may be seen as a 'badge of disability', an obvious message to society and a stigma with emotional consequences.

For those whose disability is less obvious or hidden, they may be so conscious of it that they feel that its name is branded across their forehead for the entire world to see. How confident people will feel in themselves and about themselves relates to their feelings of self-esteem and value. Loss of function, role or body image are powerful factors in self-esteem and confidence. People often say, as previously indicated, 'they do not see me, they only see the chair'. Sometimes the person sees themself as 'only a chair'.

When a disability occurs this may be accompanied by multiple changes in life including loss of independence, loss of employment, loss of status in the family or relationship (e.g. loss of the role of breadwinner) which may be taken over by the partner, thus changing the balance of the relationship. All these losses cause grief, and grieving needs to be allowed. Initially, it is difficult to see far ahead to the regaining of any independence and the possibility of a new role or job. Survival may be the all-important factor. The effect on sexual relationships may be considered a loss and major concern for some people but for others this will be further down the priority list until later, when 'reality' returns and a new pattern of life is developed. The process of loss and grieving applies not only to the person who has become disabled, but also to those close to them. Partners, too, suddenly find themselves thrust into a new role. It is very easy for the focus to be on the person who has become disabled and the needs of the partner may be overlooked. They will be trying to cope in this confusing situation and may also have fears and doubts.

Sometimes, the partner comes to see the person who has become disabled as unwell, as indeed they may be at first. Needing to carry out nursing duties, such as intimate body care, may reinforce this view and cause increased confusion over respective roles. It is a very big step to switch from nurse/carer by day to a lover by night. If the partner is perceived to be unwell it may influence the way that they are treated, or there may be a feeling of avoiding stress or putting demands on the disabled person. Unfortunately, these feelings are not often verbalised and confronted. Avoidance of making demands 'in a sexual sense' may feel like rejection and be misinterpreted as being no longer a sexual partner, desirable or attractive, reinforcing their own view of themselves as being of poor value. Body image is especially important in this context. Damage to the face, such as scarring due to laceration or burning or asymmetry due to stroke, is often particularly distressing because, of all parts of the body, the face is usually uncovered.

Although most people will acknowledge that personality is very important in a relationship, it is physical attributes that make the first impression.

---

**Case study D**

David came into the consulting room with a pronounced limp. Thirteen months previously he had a full-length amputation of his leg following a road traffic accident. The injury meant a very high amputation so that the prosthesis was difficult to fit. 'I always hope people will think I have a bit of arthritis', he said. He was devastated that anyone might realise that he had 'a limb missing', he saw this as a source of shame as he would be seen to be a lesser person.

**Case study E**

Edith showed dismay and distress when being naked exposed her deformities, due to rheumatoid arthritis, saying, 'look at me, what a mess'.

---

Self-esteem, confidence and body image influence the making of relationships and sustaining them. They have an important effect on sexual performance, which depends on both emotional and physical factors. Many people, with or without disabilities, have sexual difficulties due to emotional causes. People with disabilities appear to have no more and no less psychosexual problems than anyone else, but may have more sexual difficulties.

It is important to explore the emotional and physical factors when there is a sexual problem and disability. When there are physical difficulties there is also usually an emotional factor involved. Although counselling and exploring emotional factors may help to solve the problem these cannot replace a function that is lost due to physical damage or disease (e.g. transection of the spinal cord or demyelination in multiple sclerosis). Work needs to done about the emotional factors, but a practical approach may be needed for the physical problems (see Chapter 4). Not being 'a good catch' can result in withdrawal from the social scene and inappropriate behaviour may develop. The feelings of desperation to have a partner may mean that all opportunities or potential opportunities are grasped. For example, any interest shown by talking or having a coffee together may initiate a pattern of behaviour that can be described as 'rushing your fences' or 'taking things too fast'. Perhaps pursuing heavy chat-up lines or physical contact, lest another chance may not arise.

---

**Case study F**

Fred, a young man aged 18 years, had a road traffic accident at the age of 15 and sustained a severe head injury. He had been labelled a 'high flyer' and was aware of this. Although his accident meant he had lost his intellectual capacity, he was conscious that his peers were leaving him behind. He was desperate to have a girlfriend as they had, and 'would go for anyone from 15 to 50'.

---

Work needs to be done on exploring why there is this haste and investigate how this feels for the other person. This behaviour is often unproductive and drives people away.

## Further reading

Skrine R (ed) (1989) *Introduction to Psychosexual Medicine*. Montana Press, Carlisle.
Draper K (ed) (1983) *Practice of Psychosexual Medicine*. John Libbey, London.

# CHAPTER 4

# Practical problems: 'how to do it'

Practical sexual problems more usually arise with people with physical disability. For people with learning disability it is more often a lack of information and education that causes problems. People with an acquired disability may have already experienced a sexual relationship, so they have some expectation and experience to build on. It can be quite a shock for the person and their partner if they find that the disability has made the usual way they make love difficult or impossible. In contrast, for young people with a congenital disability they may have anxieties about whether, or how, they can have a physical relationship at all.

It is important to explore the exact nature of the physical disability. Much of lovemaking relies on desire and other emotions but in the carrying out and expressing of these feelings, there is a physical response. Damage to the blood or nerve supply can interfere with the sexual physical response. For others, it may be difficult to get into a position to make love, or there may be limitations that interfere with foreplay (e.g. the loss or impairment of hand function and sensitivity).

Although the focus often seems to be on penetrative sex, sexual intercourse, it should be remembered that 'there is more to sex than sexual intercourse'. For some couples (heterosexual or same-sex) penetration may not be possible or desired, but there are many aspects of sexual pleasuring to be explored. Touching can be a very valuable aspect of lovemaking and often for people with sensory loss (e.g. after spinal injury), other parts of the body above the lesion can become hypersensitive. This can heighten pleasure but this may be so acutely sensitive as to be painful (e.g. over-sensitive nipples). Gentle exploration is important for the couple to find out what suits them best. Oral sex can be very fulfilling for some, whereas others will find it distasteful. As for everyone, it all comes down to personal preferences.

Where there is a loss of hand function, using a vibrator can be helpful. If the hand is able to retain some grasp, but the fine movements are lost, the vibrators available in sex shops, or from FP Sales,* are suitable. It can be used as an extension of the hand and if there is some movement in the wrist or elbow, the vibrator can be used to stimulate the partner or themselves. If there are difficulties in grasping, then a more sturdy vibrator may be necessary.[1]

People with physical disabilities are usually very good problem-solvers as this skill is necessary to survive and get through the day. Although they are often embarrassed when attending to discuss sexual difficulty, it is valuable to find out what the precise difficulty is and then address the problem. It is essential to be explicit in exploring these issues. Hesitancy sometimes exists because of attitudes to being sexually active. A willingness to investigate the situation and look at options can be releasing for the patient and their partner. The climate during the consultation should be that it is both reasonable and acceptable for these needs to be addressed. If penetrative sex is what is required there needs to be an erect penis and an accessible, available vagina or rectum.

## Male problems

Many men without disability experience problems in obtaining or sustaining an erection. The causes may be emotional or physical, or often a mixture of both. Accurate diagnosis is essential and counselling is valuable. There are several practical ways to deal with this problem. All these need exploring to enable the man or the couple to make a choice.

*SexWare, PO Box 1078, East Oxford DO, Oxon OX4 5JE.

# Injections

Intracavernosal injections are available (e.g. alprostadil (Caverject)). Once injected, this results in an erection which can be sustained, often for an hour. Some couples find this inappropriate and unacceptable. Most men have anxieties about injecting into the penis. A practical difficulty can exist if the man has impairment of hand function as the injection needs to be given prior to intended lovemaking. Usually, the man is given a test dose in a clinic setting to test his response and is then taught to self-administer. If the man is unable to give the injection, his partner may be willing to do so. This situation obviously needs careful negotiation.

Users are instructed not only how to give the injection, and where exactly to inject it, but what to do should the erection be sustained for four hours. If this occurs it is important to attend for treatment to reduce the erection by aspiration of blood from the penis, or by antidote, or perhaps via surgical intervention, since penile damage can result if the erection is for more than six hours duration.

Couples are usually advised to restrict use of Caverject to once or twice a week, as fibrosis at the site of the injection can occur. Some people may find this restrictive, but for many people who have been unable to perform, once or twice a week sounds very attractive. Indeed, babies have been conceived using this method.

Two alternatives to intracavernosal injections have been available since 1998 and are discussed below.

# The urethral route

One is alprostadil (Muse) for delivery as a pellet introduced into the urethra. Although some men will have reservations about placing the pellet into the penis it appears less daunting than putting a needle in the shaft of the penis. Reports indicate that side-effects from this mode of delivery are not a major problem.[2,3] The commonest is mild penile pain but not usually of sufficient severity to wish to discontinue treatment. Only rarely were cases of priapism or penile fibrosis reported.

This would seem to be a valuable addition to the choices available. However, a prerequisite for use is that the man passes urine prior to inserting the pellet. This moistens the urethra and improves absorption of the drug and reduces the risk of urethral irritation. Unfortunately, this requisite means that this delivery route is unsuitable for those men who are unable to pass urine due to an ileal conduit. Condom usage is essential if the partner is pregnant to avoid side-effects to the foetus.

## The oral route

The second alternative is Viagra (sildenafil).[4] This has been hailed as a 'wonder drug' in the USA and is on sale over the counter there. Its sales are said to have overtaken those of Prozac (fluoxetine). This drug is now licensed in Britain and until early 1999 was available on a private prescription only, not on NHS prescription. However, in January 1999 the government proposed changes and intend to limit by law those who can receive NHS prescriptions.* This would mean men with certain conditions – multiple sclerosis, diabetes, spinal injury, single gene neurological disease – and those who have had pelvic or prostate surgery would be eligible for NHS prescriptions. Men with erectile dysfunction from other causes will need private prescriptions. These proposals are very controversial. Interestingly, it seems that many men in the USA are using it, not to treat erectile dysfunction, but to enhance sexual performance. Quick on the heels of the announcements about the drug in the lay press have come reports of death in men using Viagra. Whether these can be attributed to the drug, its misuse or sexual activity is not known. Viagra must never be used with nitrates as this combination can result in life-threatening trauma.

## Vacuum pumps

Another method to obtain an erection is the use of a vacuum pump device. As with the injection, some forward planning is necessary. Operating the pump requires two functioning hands but again, these could be those of the partner. Several types of vacuum pump are available but all are rather expensive.[5]

*In May 1999, the High Court ruled that the circular sent by the Health Secretary to GPs urging them not to prescribe was unlawful.

In essence, a vacuum is created by placing a plastic tube over the penis and using a small pump. The vacuum produced elongates the penis. A special rubber band (with side handles for easy removal) is placed at the base of the penis to sustain the erection and the plastic tube removed. Some men have used ordinary rubber bands for this purpose. However, this is potentially hazardous as the band cuts into the penis as it swells, making removal very difficult and it is especially hazardous if the man has sensory loss, as he will not be able to feel that the band is in place. Someone, either himself or his partner, has to remember that it is there and ensure its removal.

## Sex aids

Another option to enable penetrative intercourse is the use of a sex aid such as those available in sex shops or mail order. There needs to be discussion with and between the couple. Some people find the thought of using a sex aid exciting, but others are put off by it.

No one questions the use of physical aids for other purposes, for example, spectacles, sticks, hearing aids and wheelchairs, to enable or facilitate an activity. A sex aid can be included in the same category. The penis prosthesis fits over the flaccid penis and thus is larger than an erect penis. It is important to use a lubricant before penetration for it to be comfortable for the partner. Of course, sex aids should always be used according to instructions given by the manufacturer or the clinician (e.g. some aids are unsuitable for internal use).

## Implanted devices

A permanent solution for penile erection is to have a surgically implanted device. These vary from simple flexible stiffeners which means the penis can be in an erection position or down between the legs, or more complex devices with reservoirs under the abdominal skin connecting chambers implanted in the corpora cavernosa to enable erections to be produced at will. These methods need to be discussed with a urologist as they are very specialist devices. Obviously, this is an invasive method and requires surgery. Some people are willing to consider this, but for many, whose health is variable, it may not be an option they wish to choose. For example, men with conditions such as multiple sclerosis find that surgery can be a setback to their general health and it takes them longer to regain their optimal function. This occurs following any surgical intervention and would include the implantation of a device, and this is a risk that many men do not feel they can take.

## An alternative method

Where there is difficulty in obtaining a full stiff erection it is often possible to ease the semi-erect penis into the vagina using either partner's fingers. The woman may be able to aid this by drawing the penis into her vagina using her pelvic floor muscles. An increase in the erection may occur after this, but even if it does not this can still be very satisfying to both partners. This procedure is sometimes referred to as 'stuffing'.

## Female problems

For women, there are fewer options available if endeavouring to have an accessible and available vagina. Some women do not have a vagina; this may be due to surgery as treatment for disease which has necessitated its removal (e.g. with total pelvic clearance for the treatment of cancer). If babies are born without a vagina, it is usually possible to have plastic surgery later to provide a functional vagina.

For the vagina to be accessible, each partner needs to be able to get into a position such that penetration is possible (see Positions). If the difficulty is due to restricted movement because of pain (e.g. arthritis of the hip), adjusting the medication to gain maximum freedom from pain and maximum mobility can be helpful. If there is no accessible or available vagina, then the possibility of a sex aid can be considered. If possible, the woman places the artificial vagina between her thighs. As with the artificial penis it is essential that both partners are comfortable using the aid. The man is able to place his penis in the artificial vagina. It is advisable for him to use a condom as this allows easier cleaning of the aid after intercourse. By using the aid, the couple are able to experience the physical and emotional closeness of sexual intercourse. The ability to fantasise, or perhaps to be able to recapture memories from the past, can add to the pleasure. In the cold light of the consultation, aids do not usually appear attractive. However, if the clinician works with many people who may need aids, it is useful to be able to show them and allow them to handle it when discussing this option. Sometimes there are problems obtaining a sex aid, which may be due to physical difficulties (e.g. access to a sex shop), or there may be hesitancy about going into a shop or being seen going into a shop due to the somewhat sleazy reputation of these outlets.

Mail order or purchase via the Internet can be invaluable in this situation.* In fact, many retailers are very helpful to people with disabilities or to medical staff investigating the availability of suitable sex aids for the patient. Indeed, if the professional sees a number of people with these requirements, it is often useful to investigate the situation in your locality, so you are able to knowledgeably discuss this with patients when making recommendations.

## Masturbation

This is an important aspect of sexual expression and pleasure for many people, both male and female. There can be some practical problems in being able to do this. Where there is impairment of hand function or no hand function the commonest method of masturbation (i.e. manual stimulation) can be difficult or impossible. This not only includes weakness or paralysis but an inability to control the grip, which may be vice-like and become very painful.

Some people find using a vibrator valuable in this context, if there is any ability to hold it. Although often perceived as a 'woman's thing' men can experience enjoyment from stimulating the shaft of the penis with a vibrator. Other men, including those without suitable hand function, obtain satisfaction by lying on their abdomen and moving backwards and forwards. Suitably placed pillows or cushions can be helpful in this context in increas-

*SexWare, PO Box 1078, East Oxford DO, Oxon OX4 5JE.

ing friction and pressure. Some men who can manually stimulate themselves like to have an artificial vagina for increased pleasure and fantasy when masturbating.

Sometimes, because of disability, the person is unable to masturbate themselves manually or use any of the techniques mentioned above. Under these circumstances they may ask a carer to help them. This is a very emotive situation and fraught with potential problems, as it is open to misinterpretation. It places both the person with the disability and the carer in a very vulnerable position, particularly if there is impairment of understanding due to injury, disease or learning disability. This activity could be seen as exploitive and abusive. It would be very unwise for a carer to carry out this request without careful thought and discussion with senior colleagues. Ideally, there should be a policy to cover this situation, which should be implemented. When the person has a learning disability and is unable to communicate effectively, the need for help to masturbate (e.g. to relieve frustration) may be perceived by staff/carers rather than actually requested by the client. However, the client may make a direct request, as they may be physically able to masturbate but want guidance. Draft policy documents exist to cover this. Again, openness is necessary to avoid repercussions. 'Hands-on' teaching is to be avoided and the involvement of a specialist is advised (preferably using videos, illustrations and models). Only rarely, after these have been explored, is there a possibility of physical assistance. This decision should not be taken in isolation by the carer but only after discussion with the whole staff/carer team can the decision be taken. This may involve referral to the ethics committee. Of course, such discussions and the outcome must be carefully recorded. These matters are very sensitive and confidentiality within these constraints must be maintained. Other issues relating to learning disability and masturbation are discussed in Chapter 9.

## Positions

As for all couples making love, there is a need for a position that enables whatever contact is desired by the couple (this may not be penetrative intercourse), and for the position to be comfortable in both the physical and emotional sense (i.e. acceptable to both partners). There may be some limitations of position because of lack of mobility, function, or pain. For all sexually inexperienced people, disabled or not, this is a process of exploration of both individuals' needs. Couples who were making love prior to the illness or disability will have explored how they liked to do this, i.e. what was good for them. Recommencing lovemaking after an acquired disability may need an adjustment of their previous activity, and this may be affected by emotional factors.

The use of pillows can be very valuable as they can support legs that are spastic or flaccid, to enable them to retain a position and support painful joints. A pillow under the buttocks can facilitate penetration. It may be advisable to use waterproof-covered pillows in situations where incontinence can occur (see Incontinence) or if large quantities of lubricant are necessary.

As mentioned before, people with disabilities are good problem-solvers. Some couples will have worked out positions for themselves; others need support and advice. It needs to be remembered that whatever feels right for the couple and is harmful to neither is perfectly acceptable.

Many people, with or without disabilities, seem to consider that the 'missionary' position (man on top of woman) is the norm and any variation is odd or perverted. Feelings like this need to be addressed. If the man has lost confidence and self-esteem, mainly because of a major change in his role in life, to have sexual positions reversed (i.e. to be underneath) may exacerbate these feelings and this needs to be explored. David, previously mentioned in Chapter 3, who had a full-length amputation of his leg was affected by practical factors undermining his confidence and self-esteem. He had always made love in the 'missionary position'. This necessitates kneeling, which is difficult when there is one knee missing and worries about overbalancing interfered with his enjoyment. These practical problems, combined with emotional difficulties, resulted in his inability to gain or sustain an erection. He had never considered making love in any other position and was quite shocked at the thought of change. Investigation of these emotional aspects combined with practical changes in position resulted in his ability to perform again, to his great relief.

Making love does not need to be always in bed; for example,

using a chair that supports the back can be a very useful alternative. If the woman sits on the man's lap it brings the genitalia into closer contact and can allow easier access to the vagina. Sitting astride the partner in an armless chair can also be helpful. Wheelchair users may need to remove the sides for either position.

Positions that do not require weight-bearing and do not strain joints need to be discovered. One possibility is 'spoons' with both partners lying side by side with the man behind. If the woman can lean forward slightly this can make for easier penetration. Both partners' body weight will be supported by the bed. This can be particularly useful if both partners have disabilities.

When trying to facilitate finding a suitable position, it is important to consider the couple's combined abilities rather than focusing on their combined disabilities. Combined abilities can achieve results.

Positions discussed for heterosexual sex can also be adapted for homosexual sex. For a professional to address these issues is a valuable 'permission-giving' situation. Although no one has the right to give other people permission to be sexually active, or otherwise, the willingness of a professional to discuss the situation is often very reassuring.

## Incontinence

Incontinence is a problem both for people with disabilities and those without and it is embarrassing. Incontinence in some ways is associated with childhood, something that should have been 'grown out of'. It does not go with an adult sexy image and can put constraints on a relationship.

## Catheters

There is a myth that people using catheters cannot have sexual intercourse. The move towards self-catheterisation is valuable as the person can do this before making love which reduces the risk of leakage. For those with concerns about leakage, the use of a waterproof undersheet or placing towels under themselves before making love can reduce the practical problems. If there is continuous catheter drainage, this needs to be addressed.

## Catheter use in women

First, many women and their partners are uncertain where the catheter is placed in women. It is often considered 'all down below somewhere'. It must be made clear that the catheter is in the urethra not the vagina. The vagina does not have to be a 'no go area'. It is important to ascertain whether it is possible for the catheter to be spigoted, or whether continuous drainage needs to be sustained. In either case, the catheter can be taped back out of the way of the vagina and access to it. If there is continuous drainage it is important that neither partner lies on the drainage tube, as this will block drainage and also put tension on the catheter. The catheter should not be pulled, even accidentally.

## Catheter use in men

If the man has an indwelling catheter the same procedure applies, but when taping back the catheter, some leeway is needed to allow for penis erection. It should not be taped in the non-erect position as a subsequent erection will be very painful. It is advisable to lubricate the catheter from the urethral meatus, so that the penis can slide more easily along the catheter when the penis becomes erect. If not, there is trauma to the urethral mucosa. Couples often find using a condom over the penis and the catheter makes for smoother penetration. If a conveen sheath* is being used, it is possible to leave it *in situ* and remove the drainage tube and bag. The sheath can be changed later or alternatively the whole system can be removed beforehand, but this takes more time and may interrupt lovemaking. The conveen sheath has a drainage hole and is not effective as a contraceptive sheath. Although an 'indwelling' catheter can be removed entirely before lovemaking, it needs reinserting afterwards. Repeated removals and reinsertion can raise the risk of urinary tract infection. It is advisable to wash around

*Conveen sheath: a sheath covering the penis attached to a drainage tube emptying into a leg bag or bottle.

the genital area after removal of the drainage system, but this is again an interruption to lovemaking.

## Sex workers

Although for most people the desire and fulfilment of sexual activity are within a relationship, ongoing or casual, for others this is not possible or feasible. In this situation, where social contacts are limited or attempts at forming a relationship have failed, the possibility of using commercial sex services may arise. Sexual services might be the use of telephone 'Chat Lines' (these can be very expensive and can get out of hand), or correspondence of an explicit sexual nature from advertisements in newspapers, magazines or the Internet. These may satisfy sexual needs to some extent but other people will want to obtain physical sexual contact, by paying for the services of a sex worker (i.e. a male or female prostitute).

It is clearly inappropriate for health professionals to be involved in the organisation of contacts and appointments but there are important issues to be explored with the disabled person who discloses that they are considering using sexual services. It is essential to explore the risks involved, including the practice of safer sexual behaviour, to ensure that what is safe and what is risky is understood. If potentially risky activity is to occur (e.g. oral sex or vaginal or anal intercourse), advice should be given about necessary precautions (e.g. condoms or dental dam) that should be used.

When circumstances permit, the disabled person may invite the sex worker to come to their home. This can be difficult if there are other family members around but easier when living alone. Inviting a stranger into the home carries some risk, particularly if there is considerable disability, such as impaired strength or mobility. The vulnerability and risk involved is greater if the disabled person visits the sex worker at their workplace. For instance, a person who is out of his or her wheelchair and using a bed for sexual activity is less able to cope with threatening situations should they arise. In one author's (EC) experience the person using a sexual service has usually been a disabled man seeking a male or female prostitute and not a disabled woman seeking a sex worker.

Some professionals are hesitant about even discussing these issues, partly because they feel uneasy about any appearance of 'condoning' such behaviour. However, the most important factor in this is that the person considering using a sex worker's service should fully understand the inherent risks. The risks include, of course, that it might give physical gratification but will not fulfil emotional needs, athough some people have ongoing regular contact with a particular sex worker and form a bond with them. Many non-disabled people use prostitutes of either sex. This lifestyle choice is no different for a person with a disability if they have an able mind. Where there is a learning disability, the level of understanding is paramount. Not being aware of the implications would certainly rule out commercial sexual services.

# References

1.  Spinal Injuries Association (1993) *Sexuality and Spinal Cord Injury: heterosexual women.* SIA, London.

2.  Padma H, Nathan JG, Hellstrom WJ *et al.* (1997) Treatment of men with erectile dysfunction with trans-urethral alprostadil. Medicated Urethral System for Erection (MUSE) Study Group. *NEJM*, **336**: 1–7.

3.  Porst H, Abbou CC *et al.* (1996) Trans-urethral alprostadil for the treatment of chronic erectile dysfunction: the European experience. *International Journal of Impotence Research*, **8**: 131.

4.  Anon (1998) Sildenafil for erectile dysfunction. *Drug and Therapeutics Bulletin*, **36**: 81–3.

5.  Anon (1996) Pumps on test. *Health Which*, October, 177–8.

# CHAPTER 5

# Fertility

## The onset of fertility

For most young people with disabilities, whether physical or learning, puberty occurs in the same way as with everyone else; indeed, some young people will have premature onset. The appearance of secondary sex characteristics often causes alarm in the parents especially of young people with learning disability. Although there are anxieties about boys concerning sexual awareness and behaviour, the greatest anxieties occur with regard to young women. One mother said, 'when I saw the first pubic hair I flipped, I thought she would always be three. If she has pubic hair she will have periods, how am I going to cope?' She was verbalising how people with a disability, especially learning disability, are often seen as permanent children and there has been no expectation of physical and sexual development. It can be quite a shock to find that these occur.

For young women with physical disabilities, it is another difficulty to overcome. There may be practical difficulties in coping with personal hygiene and management of sanitary towels or tampons, especially if mobility is a problem or there is impaired hand function. It may be helpful to discuss the means of controlling or suppressing menstruation using hormones such as the pill or injectable contraceptives. However, it should not be assumed that coping with menstruation is unacceptable, as one young woman who was a wheelchair user said, 'I quite like to have a period and a moan about it like everybody else'.

For young women with a learning disability it can be a confusing, even frightening time. Blood usually means something bad (e.g. 'if you cut yourself you bleed'). So the issue of bleeding 'down below' can be frightening. In addition it is an unstoppable flow. After years of struggling to be continent it can be distressing and feels like a backward step. It can be helpful for young women to see that other female members of the household have periods and that the bathroom contains pads or tampons to deal with it. Some young women find it exciting and feel the need to broadcast it abroad. They sometimes produce the soiled sanitary towel in public, perhaps to 'show off', or conversely in disgust.

The practicalities of coping with menstruation need careful explanation. When, where and how often to change sanitary protection is important, to avoid leakage, soreness or unpleasant smell. Some young women do not like wearing underwear and this compounds the problem at menstruation. It may be that suppression of the period is desired. This may involve exploiting the side-effects of contraceptives (e.g. the combined oral contraceptive pill or injectable implants or IUSs). Even when there is double incontinence and the young woman has to wear incontinence pads all the time, blood loss can be an additional problem, causing distress to the young woman and her carers.

Another complication can be when young women masturbate during menstruation, as their hands can become covered with blood. This may result in smearing of blood over themselves or over other objects, or other people.

---

**Case study G**

Gayle would find her daughter and her bedroom covered in blood in the mornings. This caused little concern to her daughter, but Gayle was worried about her other daughter, aged seven, who might be distressed at the sight. In addition, it was a heavy burden to be continually cleaning up and washing everything within sight.

---

In a public place, for example, classroom or day centre, it is a difficulty for staff to maintain hygiene standards. Since the advent of

HIV and AIDS, people in general have become fearful of contamination from blood.

---

**Case study H**

Helen is 14 years old. She was referred by the community paediatric service. She has a severe learning disability and attends a special needs school. Both at home and in school Helen enjoyed masturbating. She was doubly incontinent and wore a nappy. Her hands were constantly down inside the nappy, masturbating. This activity, which clearly gave her pleasure, also occurred when she was menstruating. Her hands were then covered with blood. This became smeared over herself and her surroundings including other pupils and staff and caused considerable distress. Measures to distract Helen or reduce the incidence of her masturbating were not effective. After discussion with her parents the decision was taken to abolish the menstrual cycle and both continuous oral contraceptive pill-taking and the injectable Depo-Provera (medroxyprogesterone acetate) were considered. Her parents chose the oral method, which has proved satisfactory.

---

Dealing with inappropriate behaviour and educating or re-educating the young women is important, and the ability to offer practical help by prescribing medication is received with great relief.

## Premenstrual tension (PMT)

This syndrome is a problem for many women and can cause extremely unpleasant symptoms, including personality change and even violence which they are unable to control. These women may seek help. This problem applies equally, of course, to women with disabilities. Special problems may occur where there is learning disability. Some people with learning disability display behavioural problems and these are often exacerbated premenstrually. Some young women may become self-destructive, scratching or tearing at themselves or banging their heads on walls or windows. Another symptom may be the tendency to scream more at this time. Many women with PMT may feel like screaming but do not do so but those with moderate or severe learning disabilities may do just that. This causes distress to themselves and others. Also, some women eat inappropriately, e.g. excrement or anything that comes to hand, such as grass, paper or gravel.

---

**Case study I**

Irene, a young woman in her twenties, with severe learning disability, was known to tear at her clothes. She tore them into ribbons and if this involved scratching her skin she was impervious to the discomfort. In addition, she made howling noises. By monitoring the situation this behaviour was found to be cyclical and occurred in the seven to ten days before menstruation.

---

Careful monitoring is necessary to note whether symptoms are, indeed, premenstrual. If a correlation is found, then help is available, but behavioural problems may be sporadic throughout the cycle and thus of non-hormonal cause and they will need different treatment. There is no single answer, however, an adjustment of food intake may be very helpful since many women binge or starve themselves. Controlling food and drink intake can have striking results. A drink, some fruit, a sandwich or a meal, at two to three hourly intervals helps to maintain the blood sugar at a fairly steady level. Chocolate, often a favourite choice, should be rationed or abolished from the diet as it has a stimulating effect. Some women take evening primrose or vitamin $B_6$, which can reduce PMT symptoms. However, $B_6$ has received a bad press and has been in disrepute. This is because some women have taken excessive doses and developed toxic side-effects. There were moves made for vitamin $B_6$ to become a prescription-only medicine, in an endeavour to restrict the dose to less than 50 mg daily. However, those women who have low vitamin levels can benefit from 50 mg daily but are being warned that more than 100 mg daily may carry health risks.[1,2] Some women report benefit from magnesium supplements.

For others, the answer may be hormonal. Eliminating the menstrual cycle by taking the combined oral contraceptive pill or injectable implants or IUSs is often a very effective way of dealing with PMT. Reduction in the number of bleeds per year can be an advantage if symptoms occur in the pill-free interval, i.e. when bleeding happens. This can be achieved by tricycling (see p. 40) or, if necessary, taking the pill continuously.

Mirena, an intrauterine contraceptive system (see Chapter 6), can also be helpful in approximately 50% of PMT cases. It has been reported to JG that the remaining 50% with chronic problems can be helped by 100 mcg oestradiol patches daily together with Mirena to provide continuous protection to the endometrium (Professor Shaugn O'Brien, personal communication).

Irene disliked having periods; the bleeding seemed to distress her. Another dislike of hers was wearing pants; she would take them off whenever she could. These combined dislikes made coping with periods difficult. Without pants, blood flowed down her leg and using sanitary towels which could be stuck in her pants was impossible. With these problems it became advantageous to abolish the cycle with Depo-Provera; thus the premenstrual and menstrual problems were dealt with and she was much relieved, as were her carers.

Depo-Provera is very effective in the management of PMT. A recurrence of symptoms may occur towards the end of the injection's 'active life' when the levels are falling, but can be improved by shortening the injection interval by the equivalent number of weeks.[3,4]

If the woman requires contraception as well as an improvement of PMT symptoms, then the combined oral contraceptive pill or the injectable implant or IUS is very suitable and useful. For those where contraceptive cover is not necessary the use of Duphaston (dydrogesterone) can be helpful. This needs to be taken from days 12 to 26 of the menstrual cycle, in 10 mg twice-daily doses. However, although the *British National Formulary* states that 'this is not recommended as there is no convincing physiological basis for such treatment', it is clinically effective for some women even when there can be no placebo effect, due to severe or profound learning disability.

## To conceive or not to conceive?

Having a baby is a major life event for everyone, and the decision whether to have a baby or not is important. In an ideal world, babies would only be conceived when they were wanted, but the world is not ideal and women become pregnant for many reasons and pregnancies are not necessarily planned. However, being 'unplanned' does not necessarily mean 'unwanted', but an unplanned pregnancy can be a time of tremendous pressure and stress, not least from everybody else who seems to have an opinion. When there is a disability, society may have many preconceived ideas about parenting. This can include the attitudes of professionals – 'For many people with disabilities fear of negative judgement of professionals is a disincentive to become parents or to seek help from them'.[5] It is the professional's role to provide the woman, or couple, with information on which to base an informed decision on whether to conceive or not. A question that is often asked is whether a congenital disability will be passed on to the baby. Young people with a physical disability are usually offered genetic counselling around the time of school-leaving, and this may answer this question. Unfortunately, the offer of genetic counselling does not seem to be made to people with learning disabilities on a routine basis, so this issue needs to be addressed later in adulthood.

When it is considered that there is a risk of passing on a disability to their child, the prospective parents should deliberate very carefully. The response seems to fall broadly into two categories. Some people feel that as disabled people themselves, they are in the best position to support and advise their children on how to cope. Other prospective parents may say that under no circumstances will they take any risk of passing on their disability. Having a baby is a major decision for any couple, irrespective of whether they are disabled or not.

## Pregnancy

For some women the risks to their health of being pregnant are high. This needs to be discussed on a one-to-one basis with the physician managing the woman's healthcare. It is also important to consider what risk the woman's condition has on the pregnancy (e.g. medication being taken by the woman may affect the fetus). An advantage of forward planning is that if drugs are being taken for a condition (e.g. epilepsy) which have a teratogenic effect, then a change of medication to a drug with less risk may be possible prior to conceiving. This may need discussing well ahead of a (possibly not entirely planned) pregnancy in such couples.

Some medical conditions are exacerbated in pregnancy and others improved, but there may be a relapse after delivery. Risks and other issues concerning pregnancy and delivery should be discussed with the woman's obstetrician.

The prognosis of the disabling, progressive or life-shortening illness should be discussed, but it needs to be remembered that no individual, whether with a disability or not, knows for certain how long he or she will be around – accidents and serious illness happen. Once the decision has been made to have a baby the couple will hope to conceive when they wish. As with couples without a disability, some will achieve this, others will take longer than they would wish, and some will not conceive at all and may proceed to investigations of infertility.

Where there is a particular disability (e.g. spinal injury) that results in retrograde ejaculation or non-ejaculation, achieving conception needs medical intervention. Spermatogenesis is impaired after spinal injury. When retrograde ejaculation occurs it is possible to collect sperm from the bladder. These can be used for artificial insemination but the success rate is low. Success may be expected to improve with the increasing use of intracytoplasmic sperm injection (ICSI). Semen can be obtained by prostatic massage or electrostimulation in the rectum, the sample produced being used for insemination. Again, ICSI may be the best option. It is important to schedule insemination at the most fertile time in the woman's cycle to optimise success.

The birth of the baby is often seen as the culmination, but is in reality the beginning of a very long process of rearing a child. Focus is normally put on looking after the baby, but it needs to be remembered that this is only a fairly short, albeit demanding time and coping skills need to change through the years. For all new parents, especially first time parents, there is a period of adjustment after the birth as there are very many new skills to learn and develop.

Most people value support at this time from friends or relatives. This can be all the more important if there is a disability, and, of course, the needs of children are paramount. Where a child has parents with a disability, particularly a learning disability, there will be increased vigilance by professionals. People with a learning disability will experience many negative attitudes at the suggestion of having a baby, the fact of being pregnant, and later when the baby arrives. Many will find themselves in a position of needing to prove they can cope, as there is a risk of their children being taken into care. Ensuring that they will be able to manage and being as prepared as possible for parenting can improve their chances of success. However, they may reach the sad decision that they will not be able to cope and this requires careful exploration. It can be a soul-destroying experience to have a baby who is later taken away, and the possibility of this happening needs to be addressed.

The importance of spacing children should also be raised. It is a fact for all families that coping with more than one child is more complicated as the number increases, especially if they are born close together. By spacing the births, it is easier to manage and it may be possible to continue with the child/children in the home; whereas too many demands by more babies at close intervals can make coping difficult and may result in the children being taken into care.

Where physical health is a problem, again spacing can be important to allow recovery between pregnancies. The number of children may also need to be considered. Some couples decide on smaller families rather than push the risk to the woman's health too far. After all deliveries it is important to review these issues and to discuss safe and effective contraception to avoid an accidental pregnancy.

## Accidental pregnancy

As for anyone else, an accidental pregnancy will be a time of decision. The pregnancy may be welcomed by some, but for others it may be seen as a disaster. The same options exist as for those people without disabilities, namely, to continue with the pregnancy and rear the child, to continue with the pregnancy and place the child for fostering or adoption, or to consider termination. This is one of life's major decisions and needs to be carefully made after counselling and discussion. Although the decision must be made within time constraints, it should preferably be made without undue haste. People with physical disabilities often have able minds and will be in a position to think this through and discuss it. The factors discussed previously concerning passing on a disability, effects on the woman's health and coping with a child will need to be taken into consideration.

For people with learning disabilities, an accidental pregnancy can be a confusing situation. It is essential that this is explored carefully and explicitly using clear terminology that the person understands. Using professional jargon is in no way helpful. It is vital to work within the level of understanding of the woman or couple, which will vary tremendously depending on the degree of learning disability. Many people are able to reach a decision after careful explanation and it is extremely important that they are enabled to make their own decision and are fully involved in decision-making, because other people often try to force their views on to the woman or the couple.

In the past, decisions have been made 'for the best' with no discussion; the woman just being told, 'this is what is going to happen'. This situation can have adverse long-term sequelae.

---

**Case study J**

Julie has a moderate learning disability. When Julie was 18 she became pregnant without realising it. It was noticed that she gained weight and was taken to the doctor by her parents. A mid trimester pregnancy was diagnosed and Julie's situation was discussed by her parents, the general practitioner and the gynaecologist. Julie was not involved in these discussions but she was told she needed an operation and that it was 'for the best'. Termination of pregnancy was carried out and combined with a hysterectomy. Almost 30 years later Julie became distressed about the pregnancy and the fact that she has no children. She needed in-depth counselling to help her to deal with her emotions about the decision taken without her knowledge or consent. She found the explanation why she had never had a child, and her inability to change that, very difficult to come to terms with.

Where the woman has a severe or profound learning disability and is unable to understand or make an informed choice, the carers and professionals need to discuss the situation carefully and seek legal opinion before any termination is carried out.

Following any termination of pregnancy the future needs to be discussed. To avoid a recurrence of this situation, help in finding an effective and appropriate contraceptive must be offered if a sexual relationship is going to continue.

## References

1. Agriculture Select Committee (1998) *Fifth Report: Vitamin B6.* The Stationery Office, London.

2. Warden J (1998) Government row flares up over vitamin B6. *BMJ*, **317**: 12.

3. Cooper E (1995) The needs of people with disability. *British Journal of Family Planning*, **21**: 31–2.

4. Broome M (1992) Depo-Provera for PMT (letter). *British Journal of Family Planning*, **18**: 29.

5. Campion MJ (1995) *Who's Fit to be a Parent?* Routledge, London.

# CHAPTER 6

# Contraception

It should never be assumed that a person is infertile unless there is concrete evidence to prove it. All couples should be seen as potentially fertile until proved otherwise and unless the risk of pregnancy is acceptable, some method of contraception should be used. Assumptions are often made. It has been commonly thought that men with Down syndrome are infertile but there has been a report of a pregnancy occurring.[1]

When prescribing for people with disabilities all the usual contraindications to contraceptive methods hold. As always, there is a need for contraception to meet the person's needs, health, lifestyle and, above all, personal preference (i.e. choice is paramount). When prescribing for people with disabilities, the options are the same as for everybody else. However, the nature of the disability determines the suitability of the method on practical, medical or sociological grounds. There is a need to explore which skills are required to implement a method (e.g. manual dexterity, a good memory, mobility or agility). When faced with these problems, it often seems too complicated to find a solution, but addressing the questions: How does the disability affect contraception? and How will contraception affect the disability? helps to select options for the person to choose. It is the responsibility of the healthcare professional, as always, to give information so that an informed choice can be made by the user.

# Combined oral contraception

The first requirement for satisfactory contraceptive Pill-taking is a good memory, or for someone else (partner or carer) to have a good memory. As most prescribers know, being a 'good Pill-taker' is not a matter of intellect but of personality and lifestyle. Thus, people of high intelligence (but numerous distractions) may find it difficult to take the Pill correctly and people with a learning disability may be excellent. It is essential that clear instructions are given and possibly supervision in the early days. However, the person may be able to take on this responsibility in the long term. Once a pattern of behaviour is learnt it is often unshakeable and some learning disabled people become extremely efficient users of oral contraception. Note that **memory** may be impaired by disease or injury, for example, brain damage subsequent to meningitis or head injury or stroke, or to progressive diseases, such as multiple sclerosis.

Any disease or disability that interferes with **swallowing** will make any tablet-taking difficult. The daily crushing of the Pill is not reliable and an alternative method or route of delivery will be necessary. It must be remembered when prescribing that people with disabilities may be on other medication which may involve a large number of drugs. Each drug needs to be considered in relation to the Pill for possible interaction. The most common situation is where liver enzyme-inducing drugs are used for the treatment of epilepsy. Most of the traditional anticonvulsants such as phenobarbitone, Tegretol (carbamazepine) and phenytoin have this action. This needs to be considered in order for adequate contraception to be prescribed. Epilim (sodium valproate) and many of the newer drugs, such as lamotrigine, do not have enzyme-inducing properties. An exception is the new drug Topamax (topiramate). Whether there is any interaction needs to be considered for all drugs and reference made, as necessary, to relevant data sheets or drug information services.

Adequate prescribing of the oral contraceptive Pill where an enzyme-inducer is being used entails taking at least 50 mcg, and this dose may need to be increased to 90 mcg to avoid breakthrough bleeding. The 50 mcg Pills Ovran and Norinyl-1 are available, or a combination of 20, 30, 35 and 50 mcg Pills can be used to achieve adequate contraception. (This is not strictly within data sheet advice but is common clinical practice.) Tricycling the Pill (taking three strips end-on, without a break) reduces the risk of failure, and by shortening the Pill-free interval to four days it is possible to improve reliability. Many **post head injury** patients are prescribed anticonvulsants long term so these drugs are not used solely by people diagnosed with epilepsy *per se*. Many people with learning disability have epilepsy, particularly because of injury occurring at birth. Carbamazepine is often used for **behavioural problems** and not solely for the treatment of epilepsy. It is important to remember that when enzyme-inducing drugs are discontinued there is a delay in reduction of the enzyme-induction effect. Therefore, the use of higher-dose Pills needs to continue for two months after the enzyme-inducing drug has been discontinued before a new regime is implemented, using the usual range of 30 or 35 mcg Pills.

Another important factor is mobility – **immobility** being a risk factor for thrombosis. Any additional risk factors (e.g. smoking or obesity) make the risk of thrombosis too great and are a contraindication to taking the combined Pill.

In recent years, some women who are totally wheelchair-users have taken the combined oral contraceptive Pill, provided there are no additional risk factors for venous disease. The usual choice of Pill would be one containing norethisterone or levonorgestrel. It is usually preferable to find an alternative method of contraception, but the Pill helps by making menstruation easier to control (see below).

Any disease that causes a predisposition to thrombosis poses an increased risk when oestrogen-containing formulations are used and is thus contraindicated. Careful thought and exploration are necessary in order to find a suitable alternative method of contraception and the progestogen-only formulations are worth considering. An example of particular interest is Crohn's disease. The combined oral contraceptive Pill is a risk factor in the non-granulomatous form of Crohn's disease. If Crohn's disease is diagnosed in a Pill-taker, stopping the Pill often results in improvement in symptoms. Also to be noted is that there is an increased risk of thrombosis during exacerbation of Crohn's disease, thus making the oestrogen-containing Pill contraindicated.

An advantage for people with disabilities, either physical or learning, in using the combined oral contraceptive Pill is the control it allows over menstrual flow. Periods can be a particular problem for anyone unable to deal with the practicalities of menstrual hygiene. Sitting on soggy sanitary towels is very uncomfortable and some young women with learning disabilities are frightened by the bleeding that occurs. Bleeding usually signifies something bad, for example, injury. Distress can be caused when, after struggling to gain bladder control, this blood flow is uncontrollable. Using the combined oral contraceptive Pill allows the possibility of small planned periods ('being caught on the hop' is difficult for people with a learning disability), or having fewer periods (e.g. by tricycling or continuous Pill-taking). If breakthrough bleeding occurs this can be managed by having a withdrawal bleed for the usual length of time and then restarting the Pill.

Some people with learning disabilities adopt **unusual postures**, for example, with the legs folded beneath them almost all the time. This causes stasis in the leg blood vessels and needs to be considered when prescribing the combined oral contraceptive Pill.

## The progestogen-only Pill

The timing constraints needed for reliable contraceptive efficacy with the progestogen-only Pill mean that it is even more important to have a good memory, otherwise the contraceptive failure rate will be increased. It should also be remembered that the failure rate for methods can be of increased importance if there is a disability. However, if other medication is being prescribed, it may be possible to take the progestogen-only Pill at the same time. This can be particularly useful if there is insulin-dependent diabetes as the Pill can be taken when the insulin injection is given. Immobility is not a problem with the progestogen-only Pill as there is no increased risk of thrombosis. It is common clinical practice for people who have a past history of thrombosis to use this Pill. However, the problem of drug interaction (e.g. with anticonvulsants) remains. Increasing the dose of the Pill to two or three per day is effective in this situation but people are often advised to choose another method. The picture may be complicated for women whose weight exceeds 70 kg when, some opinions suggest, an increased dosage of the progestogen-only Pill is indicated (i.e. 2 pills a day instead of 1). Unfortunately, menstrual control is not possible with the progestogen-only Pill because it has a more variable effect on the cycle.

For all women taking oral contraception it is essential that they are well informed about how to take the Pills as failure to stick to the rules results in failure. There can be additional problems with disability. If there is impairment of vision or hearing, it is essential to check that the woman understands what to do. For example, Anne, the young blind woman mentioned previously, was prescribed a triphasic Pill by her general practitioner without being informed it was triphasic. When taking her Pill she felt for a 'full bubble' and took that pill. The pills were taken haphazardly. In a similar vein, a young deaf woman misunderstood verbal instructions and put in her diaphragm *after* sexual intercourse with the inevitable results. As always, good effective communication is essential.

## Injectables

Injectable contraception has the advantage of being effective over a period of time (8 or 12 weeks) without the need for a good memory or compliance. However, when this method is commenced it is essential to arrange follow-up so that injections are given to time – it is easy for the user to forget as the weeks pass by. There are two injectable formulations of contraception available, Depo-Provera and Noristerat. Depo-Provera is the only injectable currently licensed for long-term use or as a first-line method of contraception, but Noristerat can be used as an alternative.

Since injectables are progestogen-only formulations they have the advantage of being suitable for people who are immobile or have a past history or risk of thrombosis. An advantage of Depo-Provera is that amenorrhoea is a very common side-effect: some women have no periods from commencement, and with continued use, most women develop amenorrhoea.

If there are bleeding problems the usual management methods

are possible, which are to reduce the time interval (but not less than 4 weeks from the previous injection), or by the addition of oestrogen. If there is immobility, and thrombotic risk is present, it is important not to add the combined oral contraceptive Pill but to use natural oestrogen (e.g. Premarin, 0.625 mg or 1.25 mg) instead. This is usually sufficient to control erratic bleeding. As noted earlier, periods or other bleeding can be a problem for people with disabilities.

Many women use Pills or injectables for menstruation suppression whether or not they require contraceptive cover (i.e. they are exploiting the side-effects of the method). As with all methods it is essential that women are well informed. Depo-Provera has received bad publicity in the past, which has left myths that need to be removed by providing clear information. Many people with physical disabilities have able minds and are well able to make decisions. Where there is an impairment of understanding, it is important to provide the information in a manner that is intelligible for the user and this may often involve the carer. Concerns about weight gain are often expressed when considering using injectables. Some women do gain weight, others remain static and some even lose weight. What is clear is that some women become very hungry when using the injectable and increased food intake, especially nibbling, will lead to weight gain. Weight is an important factor in people whose mobility is impaired, who are unstable in their gait, or have painful leg conditions, where increased weight-bearing is a problem.

The slow return of fertility after stopping the injectable can be an advantage where there is a severe disability, and it is wise for there to be discussion prior to a pregnancy (i.e. forward planning). One aspect to consider is that relative oestrogen deficiency may increase the risks of osteoporosis, although this remains controversial.[2,3] Some studies indicate that there may be a problem with osteoporosis, and others that Depo-Provera is bone-trophic. Immobility is a risk factor for osteoporosis and a woman may also be taking medication, such as steroids, which increase the risk. The standard practice is to review the situation for all women who have been Depo-Provera users for five years.

Some centres measure the oestradiol level and, if this is less than 100 pg/mol/litre, advise either a change of method or addition of oestrogen. If this is given as Premarin, it will have the least possible effect on thrombotic risk. As with all other hormonal methods, there is at least a theoretical risk of reduction of efficacy if an enzyme-inducer is also being taken (e.g. some anticonvulsants). The time interval of the injection should be reduced to 10 weeks. Although no one likes injections, most people can tolerate them but some are 'terrified' of needles. An advantage for some women with spina bifida or spinal injury is that they cannot feel the needle.

Depo-Provera is very effective in the management of premenstrual tension (PMT) (see Chapter 5) and some women experience a return of PMT-like symptoms towards the end of the 12 weeks when levels are falling. This can be overcome by decreasing the time interval by the equivalent number of weeks.[4,5]

## Implants

## Norplant*

Perhaps the greatest advantage of using an implant as a method of contraception is that it is effective for five years. However, it is wise to have annual check-ups. Because of this long-term action, good memory skills and compliance are unnecessary, provided that it is remembered that at the end of five years, it will expire and efficacy will be reduced.

Being a progestogen-only method the concerns regarding thrombotic risk are reduced, as with the progestogen-only Pill and injectables. The erratic bleeding pattern which is common, especially in the first year, is a disadvantage if the practical management of bleeding is difficult for the woman. As with other progestogen-only methods, the addition of oestrogen, with the same provisos as mentioned above, is possible and may prove successful. As always, it is important that the woman is well informed and realises that bleeding is a possibility. People can cope much better if this has been addressed as part of the decision making than if they suddenly find themselves with problems.

*Norplant will be discontinued in the UK from October 1999. A very similar two-rod replacement (Zadelle) is already available in some countries.

For women with learning disability the mood swings which some users report could exacerbate behavioural problems and the practicalities of insertion and removal are important. Although insertion is not normally difficult, removal of the rods can take considerably longer. Some people with learning disability find keeping still quite difficult and would be unable to comply. If there is this problem, then it would be possible to consider insertion under a general anaesthetic, but this has attendant risks. If lying still is a problem, then it would be better to help the person to choose another method.

## Implanon

This new implant should become available in October 1999. This is a progestogen-only method releasing a steady dose of 3-keto-desogestrel over three years. Clinical trials have shown it to be very effective in preventing pregnancy (2300 women, with 73 000 cycles and no pregnancies reported).[6] In addition, there are two main advantages for all women but which are of particular use for women with disabilities. First, the incidence of amenorrhoea is higher than for Norplant (Implanon 20%, Norplant 5%), but irregular bleeding remains a possibility for some women. Secondly, as Implanon is a single rod, pre-loaded into a sterile disposable applicator, it is easier and quicker to insert and remove. This widens the choice for those who find it difficult to cope with longer procedures.

## Copper IUD including Gynefix* and IUS

One advantage of these devices is that 'they are always there', so that contraceptive cover is continuous and no compliance is needed. Another advantage is that newer IUDs have a licence for 5–10 years. Until the availability of the injectable, for women with poor memories, the intrauterine device (IUD) was an ideal method. For the woman with a disability there are two major disadvantages of using an IUD: (1) the increase in menstrual flow,

*Gynefix is a frameless implantable copper IUD first marketed in 1998.

which may mean longer as well as heavier periods, making the periods harder to manage; and (2) difficulties relating to insertion. Problems with increased flow can be overcome by the use of the Mirena intrauterine system (IUS) where the effect of the local release of progestogen is to suppress blood loss. The woman would need to be aware that there may be erratic bleeding, especially in the first year, but this will usually improve and settle. It then is a very popular option, especially because of oligoamenorrhoea, which is the norm.

More difficult may be the practicalities concerning insertion of the IUD/IUS. It is important for the practitioner performing the insertion to be able to have a good view of the cervix and to be in a position to carry out the fitting requirements accurately. In addition, it is important that the woman is in a comfortable position and able to lie still. However, with ingenuity, it is usually possible. If the woman is informed of what is required of her she will be able to address any difficulties and explain her own problems (e.g. she does not have control of her legs), perhaps due to multiple sclerosis or cerebral palsy, or is unable to abduct the hips due to arthritis. Asking about the position she uses for intercourse may be useful in finding a mutually convenient position. As always, of course, it is essential that the practitioner fitting the device is qualified.[*]

Precautions are necessary if the woman has a spinal injury. Stimulation of the cervix may cause autonomic dysreflexia, which results in a dramatic rise in blood pressure. This is an emergency situation. It would be unwise to consider fitting an IUD without medical back-up to deal with this (i.e. in a hospital centre, not a community clinic or general practitioner's surgery). It may well be that an alternative method is the better choice. For women with learning disabilities, the problem may be apprehension or difficulty in keeping still. The degree of learning disability and of understanding will be an influencing factor. If the young woman is fully mature sexually, but in other aspects much younger, it may be inappropriate to implement such a procedure without considering using a general anaesthetic. But this has other risk factors.

[*]The qualification is: Letter of Competence in Intrauterine Techniques, awarded by the Faculty of Family Planning and Reproductive Health Care, RCOG.

It is possible to build up trust with the young woman and if there is continuity of the doctor–patient relationship, it is possible to carry out IUD checks and, as maturity develops, even to change a device without a general anaesthetic. The same constraints regarding position and keeping still apply to the IUS. When discussing fitting a device in a woman who has a disability, such as rheumatoid arthritis, it needs to be borne in mind that she may need to take her medication prior to the insertion to enable greater mobility of her hips at the time of insertion. This may, of course, also be invaluable in controlling any post insertion discomfort. In the past, it was considered that for women taking oral long-term steroids it would be a contraindication to use an IUD because of perceived infection risks. However, the United States Food and Drug Administration no longer consider this a contraindication, unlike the more profound immunosuppression in the early management of organ transplantation where the concern about infection risk *is* valid.

## Diaphragms and caps

The skills required for using a diaphragm or cap are:

- some degree of manual dexterity
- the ability to get into a suitable position to insert it
- to remember to have it available and inserted when required (i.e. there is a degree of forward planning).

Diaphragms and caps, especially when the spermicide is applied, can be quite slippery objects and manoeuvring can be difficult if hand movements are impaired (e.g. by neurological damage or disease), or restricted by pain. It is easier if the user has two functioning hands, one to part the labia and the other to insert the diaphragm or cap. It is possible to fit the device with one hand but it is more difficult and leaves no hand available to 'hold on' if physical stability is a problem.

Most women are taught to insert the device by standing on one leg or squatting. These positions can be difficult if there is impaired mobility. It is possible to insert the cap lying down, but this can be a problem especially if the arms are short and hands are small (e.g. in achondroplasia). Some women insert the device by sitting (e.g. on the edge of a chair) if that is possible. Endeavouring to fit the device while sitting on the toilet can be hazardous if the cap is dropped! In these situations, it may be possible and acceptable for the device to be inserted by the partner, and this may need negotiation as both partners need to feel comfortable about this. If there is a lack of sensation then it can be difficult to know if the cap is correctly in position and this may cause loss of confidence in the method. If the device is incorrectly fitted and is, for instance, pressing too hard on the bladder neck, it may increase the risk of urinary tract infection. The efficacy of female barriers (being only 94%, range 92–98%, in the first year of 'perfect use') is also a consideration, especially in women under 35 years of age.

Forward planning improves successful management of this method. Getting into a regular routine of inserting it so that protection is there when needed is the least intrusive way to use a diaphragm or cap. Having to break off lovemaking to insert the device is intrusive and can lead to incorrect fitting or not using it at all, so the failure rate will inevitably rise! For many people with physical disabilities forward planning is necessary in most areas of their lives to get through the day, and including the insertion of the diaphragm or cap into their routine is acceptable.

For people with a learning disability forward planning is not such a pronounced part of everyday living and it may be difficult for them to use this method. It will obviously depend on the personality and level of disability. However, as mentioned earlier, learned behaviour can be unshakeable and very reliable, but consideration of using the cap or diaphragm needs careful exploration. The partner should not be neglected in this as 'two heads are better than one'.

## Condoms: male and female

Condoms are important as they have the advantage of protecting against sexually transmitted infection (STI) in addition to contraception. They are a valuable adjunct to other methods of contraception as in the practice of 'doubling up' or 'Double Dutch' (another method for contraception plus condom for STD prevention). Condoms are essential for the practice of safer sex.

Two functional hands are a decided advantage when using the condom and one partner needs manual dexterity. Putting on the condom can become part of foreplay. Putting in the female condom (Femidom) is easier to do with two hands, but can be inserted with one. It needs to be remembered that if you only have one hand for everything you become very skilled with it.

For reliability, it is essential that clear instructions are given for using this method. This is even more important if the person has a learning disability. Sometimes people are shown how to use a male condom on a banana, cucumber, broom handle or the fingers. This can be very confusing. Many people with learning disability are very literal, especially if they are autistic, and may believe that this is where it has to be put – not helpful or effective! A life-like model that resembles the erect penis, such as the Brook or Family Planning Sales model, is invaluable in this context. Discussion with the partner to negotiate using a condom is an important issue to be addressed. Everybody using condoms should be provided with information concerning emergency contraception and where to obtain it.

# Natural methods of contraception*

Some couples prefer to use natural methods of contraception for a variety of reasons – religious, cultural or a desire for using something natural and physically unintrusive. It is essential that this method is clearly understood and good teaching is necessary or the failure rate of the method rises. As mentioned before, the failure rate can have even greater importance if there is a severe disability. For reliable use it needs two people who are both committed to this method, and specially trained teachers should be consulted. These may be specialists, in particular, family planning nurses with additional training in this method, or teachers trained by Fertility UK.

*Avoiding intercourse or unprotected intercourse on identified fertile days of the cycle.

If the natural method is used by a couple prior to a disabling accident it may subsequently be unsuitable, at least in the short term, as the menstrual cycle may be disrupted and it is more difficult to monitor fertility. Many women with a spinal injury will develop amenorrhoea or an erratic cycle in the early months. Using this method when the cycle is not regular makes it unreliable. The level of understanding and application needed for this method, as it is rather complicated, means that it is usually **not** suitable for a couple with learning disability. (One author, EC, has not found it useful for such couples, and although taken publicly to task over not recommending it to people with learning disabilities, still feels it is inappropriate.)

The advent of the contraceptive device, Persona, has heralded a new advance. This device enables a couple to identify the woman's most fertile days in the menstrual cycle by testing her urine. They are advised to abstain on those days or use other contraception, e.g. condom. Results from the trials were very encouraging, but there are reports from the media that its use by the general public, who did not have the more detailed instruction about the method (as did those in the clinical trials), results in the failure rate being higher and thus less acceptable. But even **consistent** use of this method is estimated as leading to at least six failures per 100 users in the first year.[7]

## Sterilisation: male and female

Sterilisation is a major decision for everyone and needs careful thought and discussion, as it should be considered to be both permanent and irreversible. It is a commonly held view that it is possible to change your mind and 'have it reversed'. This is difficult, often not successful and, in the current climate, rarely available on the NHS.

Sterilisation is often suggested if there is a severe degree of disability or if the risks of pregnancy are high for the woman. It is important to discuss this at some length so that the couple are in a position to decide what the risk means for them (i.e. they can make an informed decision). Many severely disabled women realise the hazards of pregnancy and decide not to embark on a pregnancy, but feel unable to make the final step to sterilisation. They need very good effective contraception, which is reversible so that they feel that they have the **option** to become pregnant 'like everybody else' if they so choose, even if they know they will not do so. They may never decide to have sterilisation or may need some years to make the decision. This is where the modern intrauterine devices and systems can be particularly useful (e.g. Gyne-T 380/Gynefix/Mirena).

Women need to consider that being sterilised will stop concerns about becoming pregnant but will not have any effect on menstruation. Indeed, if a woman has been using hormonal contraception to abolish or control blood loss, she will need to continue taking these drugs after the operation or cope with menstruation again. It was hoped that endometrial ablation would be valuable in this context. Endometrial ablation in itself cannot be considered to be contraceptively safe, but in conjunction with sterilisation would be effective. However, the incidence of bleeding following endometrial ablation can be a problem, as it is difficult to ensure that every fragment of endometrium is ablated. Those that remain may bleed.

The decision regarding sterilisation for people with learning disability is a particular problem. It is essential that there is understanding for informed consent to be given. Assumptions are often made and pressure brought to bear to deal with worries around pregnancy and parenting. Parents or professional carers may raise this option. It is important that this is explored in depth so that the anxieties, needs and rights of all concerned are addressed. There are both ethical and legal aspects to this decision. It is essential that the person with learning disability is involved in the decision as much as possible. Sterilisation has been carried out on young people under the age of 18 (i.e. minors)[8] but no person is in a position to consent on behalf of someone over 18 and it is important that legal opinion is sought and the situation fully explored.[9,10] In practice, with the wide range of contraception available, sterilisation can be avoided and the risks and benefits of ongoing contraception for all of the person's reproductive life considered. It would be illogical to carry out sterilisation and then discover that the young woman needed to take hormones to control problems with menstruation. It needs to be remembered that sterilisation only deals with fertility and that people that are sterilised will still need to practise safer sex and use condoms for prevention of sexually transmitted diseases. In addition, sterilisation does not solve problems concerning vulnerability and exploitation or the difficulties of menorrhagia or premenstrual tension. Before the final decision, counselling must be given that newer methods of contraception are at least as effective and some have additional benefits.

## Emergency contraception

Ideally, information about the existence of emergency contraception should be given to all people of reproductive age. Information about what it is and where to get it should be available for all. Of course, the emphasis should be on its use for emergencies and not as a routine method. It is useful for home managers of group homes in the community to be aware of the existence of emergency contraception, so that if approached by one of their residents in a crisis situation, they can access help quickly.

Emergency contraception is available in two forms: (1) by taking Pills within 72 hours; or (2) inserting an IUD within five days of the earliest ovulation. Emergency contraception is available from GPs, family planning clinics and some accident and emergency departments. For the prescriber, it is important to remember that those women taking liver enzyme-inducers (e.g. some anticonvulsants) need an extra dosage of emergency contraceptive Pills to be effective. Instead of $2 \times 50$ mcg combined oral contraceptive Pills or Schering PC4 repeated in 12 hours, they require $3 \times 50$ mcg Pills repeated in 12 hours.

There are some women in whom the use of oestrogen-containing Pills is contraindicated and they may be reluctant to have an IUD fitted. There is a recognised alternative to be discussed using a progestogen-only formulation. To date, this method has not received approval from the Medicines Control Agency, but it is used in current clinical practice. This situation is very likely to be regularised by 2000 with the approval of a licence. This was studied by WHO in 1998 using two doses each of 0.75 mg levonorgestrel (equivalent to 20 tablets Neogest or 25 tablets

Microval or 25 tablets Norgeston) taken at 12-hourly intervals and commenced within 72 hours of intercourse.[11] Efficacy was reported as greater, and the side-effects were less, than the Schering PC4 method. This situation will be improved by the availability of 750 mcg tablets (Postinor-2) which would replace the high number of tablets required previously.

# References

1. Sheridan R (1989) Gonadal function in Down Syndrome subjects. *J Med Genet*. **26**: 294–8.

2. Cundy T, Evans M, Roberts H *et al.* (1991) Bone density in women receiving depot medroxy progesterone acetate for contraception. *BMJ*. **303**: 13–16.

3. Gbolade BA *et al.* (1998) Bone density in long-term users of depot medroxy progesterone acetate. *Br J Obstet & Gynae*. **105**: 790–4.

4. Cooper E (1995) The needs of people with disability. *Br J Fam Plan*. **21**: 31–2.

5. Broome M (1992) Depo Provera for PMT [letter]. *Br J Fam Plan*. **18**: 29.

6. Croxatto MB and Makarainen L (1998) The pharmacodynamics and efficacy of Implanon™: an overview of the data. *Contraception*. **58** (Suppl): S91–7.

7. Bonnar J, Flynn A, Freundl G *et al.* (1999) Personal hormone monitoring for contraception. *Br J Fam Plan*. **24**: 128–34.

8. Case of 'Jeanette', Lord's Appeal (1987).

9. Gunn MJ (1991) *Sex and the Law: a brief guide for staff working with people with learning difficulties* (3rd edition). Family Planning Association, London.

10. McK.Norrie K (1991) *Family Planning Practice and the Law*. Dartmouth, Aldershot.

11. WHO (1998) Randomised controlled trial of Levonorgestrel *v* YUZDE regimen of combined oral contraceptive pill for emergency contraception. *Lancet.* **352**: 428–33.

## Further reading

Belfield T (1999) *FPA Contraceptive Handbook.* FPA, London.
Guillebaud J (1999) *Contraception: your questions answered.* Churchill Livingstone, Edinburgh.
Guillebaud J (1998) *Contraception Today.* Martin Dunitz, London.
Guillebaud J (1997) *The Pill.* Oxford University Press, Oxford.
Loudon N, Glasier A and Gebbie A (1995) *Handbook of Family Planning and Reproductive Healthcare.* Churchill Livingstone, Edinburgh.
SPOD (1990) *Contraception for People with Disabilities.* Leaflet No 9. SPOD, London.

# CHAPTER 7

# Young people's special needs

Sex is high on the agenda for most young people. Adolescence can be a difficult time and there may be anxiety about self-image and how teenagers are perceived by others, most particularly their peers. This is a time when there is a great desire to be 'like everybody else', where to be different is anathema, but simultaneously there is a need to be one's self and unique, special.

These anxieties occur amidst a plethora of mixed, often chaotic, emotions in response to hormonal changes. This situation of hormonal development occurs for all young people, male or female, disabled or non-disabled. Most young people have doubts and want to be attractive, desirable, valuable, valued and loved. Worse than feeling unloved is to feel unlovable. If these issues arise for most young people, they can also apply to the young disabled.

## Physical disability

A particular problem for people with physical disabilities can be the feeling of being different which may be all too obvious if the disability is evident by loss of function (e.g. need for a stick, wheelchair, need for signing or visual impairment). The body image as perceived by themselves or others, or as projected, has an important effect on self-esteem. Some young people may hide their disability and endeavour to deny it exists. This can lead to problems if this causes deterioration in the level of care (e.g. neglecting the management of cystic fibrosis). Conversely, less obvious or hidden disability, such as deafness or memory loss after head injury, can be a problem often resulting in feelings of isolation as no consideration may be given to their particular need.

It should be noted that even in institutions, such as residential schools or colleges, where everyone is an individual but has a common factor of disability, anxieties around these issues of desirability and attractiveness, of being valuable and valued, remain important. Peer pressure is felt very much by the resident students. As in all enclosed establishments, anxiety about confidentiality and gossip exist to worsen the problem.

For young people in mainstream schools the feeling of being different may be more marked. It has been noted by staff undertaking sex education in classes including non-disabled and disabled students that for the most part, the disabled young people appear to feel that it is irrelevant to them, and do not take any active part in discussions. It may be, of course, that this subject is too difficult or painful for open discussion.

There may be an underlying lack of knowledge or understanding, not only about the content of sex education talks but about what the particular disability means as regards a sexual relationship. How much activity and performance is possible, or are some activities impossible, due to the disability and resulting loss of function? Although there may be concerns about genetic risk, there is a much higher interest at this stage in sexual performance. Anxieties around passing on inherited diseases or disabilities tend to come later.

If the young person feels doubtful and wants information about sexual matters, it may be difficult for them to access this information or services, not only because of physical constraints but because there are worries about who to ask (peers, teachers, health professionals or parents?). How will these requests be received? What sort of language should they use? Will the young person and those approached be too embarrassed? Will they shock the person they are asking? Will the request be ignored, laughed off or made public knowledge with the attendant feelings of rejection, and maybe humiliation, or will it be accepted and valued as a reasonable request or anxiety?

## Parents and carers

If most teenagers are endeavouring to find and establish their own identity, most parents are wondering and worrying how to cope with it, how far, when and how to 'let go'. This can exacerbate the so-called generation gap, an anxious time for parents as well as for young people. This situation is often worsened if the young person has a disability. The usual loosening of constraints and taking on of responsibility for themselves can be difficult if some elements of personal care need to be continued by the parent. If most parents are concerned for the welfare and well being of their children as they become adults, this is even more marked for parents of young people with disabilities who may find it difficult to let go. The parents may fear the reaction of society to the young person, the letting go process becomes more difficult and, as a result, may become more protective. Many teenagers perceive their parents' attitude and actions as restrictive and their protectiveness as irksome. For a young disabled person these feelings may be much stronger. There is often a great deal of anger concerning their disability and, moreover, the protectiveness of the parent or carer seems to be smothering.

## Working with parents

Many parents of young people with disabilities feel anxious not only on behalf of the young person but also about how they are going to cope themselves. Often the attitude of other people towards parents of teenagers is unhelpful, fortifying the 'disabled people don't do that' myth.

Opportunities to provide help and support need to be taken up. There are often feelings of isolation and the support of other parents who have experienced this phase, or who are experiencing it, can be very helpful.

Health professionals and schools need to be prepared to respond effectively to queries raised and to be prepared to raise the issues themselves. Accurate information is very helpful in defusing anxiety. Some special needs schools in Hampshire are working together to produce information leaflets on such topics as menstruation, for parents to be able to share with their daughters. These provide accurate information and highlight situations where help can be sought (e.g. the management of periods or premenstrual tension). Many parents feel 'stuck with' problems and are unaware that help is at hand. Similarly, parent group meetings where there may be a speaker and group discussion can be useful. Some organisations for specific disabilities, such as the Down's Syndrome Association, can supply information and guidance concerning problems relating to a specific disability. Often, just knowing that others have similar problems and that there may be ways of dealing with them is reassuring.

A one-to-one consultation to address the problems of the individual young person can explore difficulties and options for management. If the young person is so severely learning disabled that they are unable to take a real part in the discussion, and become bored and restless, it is initially more effective to discuss the situation and options with the parents and carers without the young person being present. A more effective discussion with the teenager can take place later when the salient points have been clarified. Talking about some practical issues like menstruation can open the door to discussing more sensitive issues, such as sexuality and its expression.

Even if independence has been gained and the 'child' is living a separate life away from home, the situation can change with the advent of an acquired disability (e.g. after a road traffic accident or debilitating degenerative disease) where the capacity to live independently is, at least temporarily, lost. This sometimes means a move back into the family home and the parent takes on the role of carer, and perhaps having to undertake personal functions such as toileting, that had ceased many years before. The child–parent role is then reinstated. This can be difficult for both, especially as embarrassment may accompany intimate body care. In addition, this vulnerable period of undermined self-esteem, the loss of independence, can be frightening, disillusioning and undermining in the need to find a new identity. After all, the former personality is there within, only the external 'shell' may be different: 'She or he treats me like a child' is a common comment.

## Learning disability

For the young person with a learning disability, adolescence may be an even more confusing time. The hormonal changes that occur in all young people also occur in those with disabilities. However, there may not be the capacity to understand what is happening, why they feel differently, or moody, etc., and perhaps have no words to express these feelings.

Body changes may not be noticed or may become the source of increasing interest. This can result, for instance, in inappropriate behaviour (e.g. masturbating at inappropriate times or in inappropriate places). It is at this stage that it is necessary for patterns of appropriate behaviour to be addressed. If no one explains to the young person that masturbating in the street or in the supermarket is inappropriate, then the behaviour will continue, often with punitive results. It is important that the young person knows that it is 'OK' and natural to want to masturbate, but it must be in an appropriate place and this means privacy. Otherwise, many negative messages can be received if 'a slapped wrist' or 'don't do that, it is dirty' message is given. There are many old wives' tales about masturbating which threaten catastrophe, such as blindness or madness. These myths still abound and are very unhelpful, to say the least. If no one gives guidelines as to how to behave with the opposite sex, once again inappropriate behaviour may occur and become established. To give an example, women do not take kindly to having their breasts grabbed by strangers in the street. This causes distress, and consequences, for both the woman and the person with learning disability who may be completely unaware of how unacceptable this behaviour is, and dismayed at the distress caused.

**Case study K**

Karl, a young man with moderate learning disability, wanted to be everyone's friend. He was intrigued by women's breasts and could not resist

> touching them in the street or wherever he happened to be. He had not thought about this, but when questioned, assumed that the woman would enjoy this as much as he did. He thought it was normal behaviour. He was shocked at the reaction to his behaviour and felt misunderstood.

If patterns of behaviour are established early many problems can be avoided when the person is older, when society is less tolerant. Inherent in this is the concept of personal space. Everyone needs to understand, as far as possible, that everybody has the right to call their body 'their own', and that no one has the right to invade that person's body or personal space. Where physical contact may occur, especially of a sexual nature, both participants must be in agreement. If either party dissents, then touching is not acceptable and becomes abusive if persistent. It is important that the young person is aware that they do not have to accept anyone touching them, that they can say no, if necessary reinforced by gesture, or if there is no speech available to them, by clearly indicating **no**, with body language, from the outset.

## The professionals' role in reducing vulnerability

With respect to the vulnerability of the young learning disabled person it is essential that professionals who need to touch or examine the teenager ensure that they make it clear who they are and why they are behaving in this way. This applies whether they are a doctor, nurse, physiotherapist, occupational therapist or carer. For some examinations or care, intimate touching may be necessary and this needs to be clearly explained. Without this clarity, the young person is vulnerable to exploitation and abuse by any one who suggests that they lie down and take their clothes off.

As regards social contact, the professional needs to be supporting appropriate safe patterns of behaviour in the young person. In the past, over-familiar behaviour has been accepted from people with learning disability (e.g. hugging or kissing strangers on a first meeting). This behaviour would not be tolerated from a person without a learning disability, it would be decreed inappropriate. Failure to discourage this familiarity, of course in a kind non-rejecting way, by perhaps offering to shake hands, perpetuates behaviour and makes that person very vulnerable. It may be safe for the person with the learning disability to hug **you**, but some strangers may be abusers. It is the responsibility of us all to help vulnerable people to be safe.

## Parents and carers

People with disabilities, especially learning disabilities, are often seen as children and asexual or non-sexual. Coming to terms with his or her burgeoning sexuality can be especially difficult if you perceive your child as remaining in a permanent state of child-hood. The need to be protective, and having an awareness of the pitfalls of life and his or her vulnerability make 'letting go' all the harder.

When talking to parents about their children their common anxieties were:

- exploitation and abuse

- where to draw boundaries

- how to cope with adolescent mood swings

- how to cope with inappropriate sexual behaviour.

For parents of girls there were worries around coping with periods and the risk of pregnancy. Anxiety about catching an 'infection' was a concern of all the parents. For those parents whose children were biddable the anxiety was greatest. There was some relief among those parents whose children shunned contact, as they felt it was one less problem. There was a dichotomy of feeling between 'wanting the best out of life', which included rela-tionships, but fear of the consequences of becoming close to another. There may also be fears about being emotionally hurt. Unfortunately being hurt is part of the highs and lows of relation-ships in life, and being overprotective limits life's experience. Sometimes in a bid to seek independence and break from such overprotectiveness, young people move into marriages as a means of escape, sometimes in undue haste and with unfortunate consequences, including abuse.

Feelings of self-doubt and lack of confidence may mean that the young person is non-selective about relationships and that even the slightest interest from someone will be grasped in case no one else shows interest. This, again, lays the young person open to being taken advantage of. Understandably, those young people with life-threatening or life-shortening diseases are anxious to grasp every opportunity and to 'pack it all in while I have the chance'.

## Further reading

Barnardos (1993) *Meeting the Personal and Sexual Relationship Needs of Children and Young Adults with a Learning Disability.* Barnardos, London.

Docherty J (1986) *Growing Up: a guide for children and parents.* Modus Books, London.

Muskett K (1995) *A Simple A to Z of Sex: a guide for young adults with speech and language impairments.* AASIC, London.

Stenager WL (1995) Sexual problems in young patients with Parkinson's disease. *Acta Neurologica Scandinavica.* **91**: 453–5.

SPOD (1990) *Sex and Your Child with a Disability.* Leaflet No 7. SPOD, London.

# CHAPTER 8

# Some specific disabilities

So far this book has considered general issues concerning sexuality and disability. Against a background acknowledging that each person is unique, each disability needs to be addressed individually. This chapter discusses some more specific problems that may apply to certain disabilities.

## Cardiovascular problems

After a heart attack or stroke the common anxiety is that sexual activity will, because of increased physical activity and stress, cause a relapse or further heart attack or stroke. When talking to groups of couples, where one partner has had a heart attack, they were concerned about when to resume sexual activity and what they were 'allowed' to do. Information is sometimes given, usually in the form of a leaflet, but there was often a reluctance to ask these questions of staff, who were also hesitant to raise the issue. Also, it was often a taboo subject between the couple. In general, the advice needs to be, 'when you feel ready to begin making love and certainly if you are able to walk a flight or two of stairs without problems'. There must be a proviso that if any symptom, such as chest pain, occurs the activity needs to be curtailed and it should not, at least at first, be too athletic. Less active, gentle sexual activity is valuable and therapeutic and often less stressful than avoiding sexual activity. Frustration can raise the blood pressure too!

One of the authors (EC) was involved with a study group organised for people who had experienced a heart attack and their partners. 'Sex After Heart Attack' was the topic for discussion. It was the partners of men who had a heart attack who were most worried lest their partner have another heart attack during intercourse. These fears of making demands on their partner and the thought of subsequent guilty feelings were inhibitory. Most of the men, however, held a different view, saying 'It's a good way to go, on the job'. But they then acknowledged that they had not thought of this situation from their partner's point of view.

---

**Case study L**

Lloyd, a man in his forties, had noticed that his beta-blockers had affected his performance and interfered with his ability to have an erection. His way of dealing with this was not to take his medication if he wanted to make love. Obviously, this is not the right way to deal with this problem. His wife was frantic knowing he had not taken his medication and was afraid 'he would die during sex'. They did not discuss it and he had no idea of the level of anxiety she was experiencing on his behalf.

---

Problems concerning performance and medication need to be addressed by the prescriber. Returning to sexual activity is one more step on the way back to normal living.

Following a stroke or subarachnoid haemorrhage, patients and partners will have similar anxieties to those experienced after heart attack. In addition, in patients who have experienced a stroke there may be changes in personality or emotional instability may occur (see Chapter 3). Practical difficulties may arise as a result of loss of function (e.g. hemiparesis), and then the more specific issues, such as positions, need to be explored (see Chapter 4).

## Musculoskeletal problems

Any condition that restricts movement can interfere with sexual performance, not least in the ability to get into a suitable, comfortable position to make love. Weight-bearing can be a particular problem because of pain or fragility (e.g. fragile bone syndrome, osteogenesis imperfecta). The most common medical condition causing problems in this respect is arthritis – **osteoarthritis** and **rheumatoid arthritis**. Both conditions result in problems with mobility and pain. Making love is not much fun if there is pain. So there can be combined problems of being unable to move and any attempted movement being painful. Pain is in itself debilitating but rheumatoid arthritis, in particular, is a generalised debilitating disease and may have a marked effect on sexual relationships or the desire to be sexually active. In addition to the limitations of mobility and pain rheumatoid arthritis produces deformities of joints and in this way affects body image and has a secondary emotional impact which itself needs to be recognised and addressed (see Chapter 3).

Painful hands may make touching or caressing a partner clumsy, difficult, or impossible. A sex aid may be helpful but an attempt to control, reduce, or abolish the pain is a distinct advantage. An adjustment in the time of taking medication to obtain maximum mobility and freedom from pain is valuable, as is the use of pillows to support painful joints. Utilising the best time of day to make love, if appropriate and convenient, will lessen the problems of feeling debilitated.

Assumptions are sometimes made by professionals that people over a 'certain age' will not be affected by sexual difficulty because they are 'past it' anyway. This is an assumption that should never be made – the oldest man in EC's sexual difficulty clinic was 87 years old. What the effect is for any particular person or couple is what is important. Indeed, many young people have joint problems, arthritis is not a disease affecting solely older people. Young people may need and want help but find it difficult to ask in a situation where most others in the clinic are older.

## Neurological problems

Neurological disabilities may be congenital or acquired, subsequent to trauma or disease.

# Congenital

An individual assessment needs to be made as to the specific effects of the congenital disability, which depends on which nerves are affected. For example, for a person with **spina bifida** the level and degree of the lesion will affect the degree of disability. Some people experience loss of sensation, which is important in receiving touch in sexual pleasuring. The site of the lesion will affect the capacity to have an erection or ejaculate. Some men may experience retrograde ejaculation.

# Head injury

The site and severity of the head injury will both affect the degree of disability following head injury. It will therefore have varying effects on behaviour and impairment of function. There may be additional injuries from the accident that also contribute to the outcome. Initially, it may be that 'survival is all', but later, as conscious levels improve, there will be increasing awareness. The situation usually changes considerably over time and the final recovery outcome may not be apparent for months or years.

From the person's point of view the greater the severity of the injury, the less the level of awareness of what has happened. With improving levels of awareness the effect of the accident will be perceived with attendant emotional and practical consequences.

Patients recovering from severe head injury may display blatantly sexual behaviour, due to disinhibition. This may be self-display, for example, nudity, inappropriate masturbating or sexual advances towards others, relatives, friends, staff or members of the public. This can be quite indiscriminate. Distress is often caused to the relatives who will contrast this disinhibited behaviour with the person's usual behaviour and be embarrassed on their behalf. They know how distressed the person would be if they realised how they were behaving. This heightened sexual awareness may only be a phase in recovery but for others it is permanent. Dealing with this, either on a temporary or permanent basis, is stressful for all concerned except possibly the patient. Behaviour can be considered inappropriate if it causes offence or distress. The problem must be addressed in discussion with the patient.

---

**Case study M**

Malcolm, a man in his forties, suffered a severe head injury several years ago. His sexual interest is high and this is fuelled by his desire for a partner. He endeavours to fulfil this need by lunging at every woman who comes within arms length (i.e. family, care staff or any visitor), indiscriminately. As can be imagined, all women have been warned and walk around him just beyond 'grabbing distance' as a means to avoid him. This, of course, has increased his level of frustration and also of isolation. Apart from 'telling him off' no one discussed with him why he did it, or the effect his behaviour was having. It was necessary to explore his feelings and how counter-productive his behaviour was in achieving his goal. He needed to be able to appreciate that it was not his physical appearance and his need to use a wheelchair that drove women away, but his behaviour towards them.

After counselling Malcolm was able to understand how counter-productive his behaviour was, and why, but he found it very difficult to implement change. In part, this was due to his high level of frustration and also due to his memory loss, which necessitated constant reminders. With the help of his carers he continues to gain some control over his situation.

---

People deal with inappropriate approaches in different ways. Staff may for instance laugh it off, which can sometimes feel like a put down, use the slapped wrist technique which is punitive, or become offended. Variation in response is very confusing for the patient as mixed messages are received. There needs to be a common response in this situation. Often the problem is not addressed with the patient who may wonder why everyone is avoiding him or her. A simple explanation within the level of understanding is needed. This may need to be accompanied by action (e.g. removal of the wandering hand), and to be repeated many times especially when there is a short-term memory impairment. The eventual outcome may range from no interest in sex at all to an obsession with sex and all shades in between.

It can be difficult for the partner to know how to deal with this situation. Where there is loss of language partners are often concerned as to how their head-injured partner feels about sex and whether advances are wanted or not. In this situation relying on body language or response may be the only way to assess this.

---

**Case study N**

Naomi said that she felt very uneasy because she could not communicate with her husband. She loved him and felt that having a sexual relationship was normal as being part of their marriage and thus a return to some semblance of everyday life as it was before the head injury. His lack of indication to her made her feel inhibited in making love to him as it felt like abuse. This caused her considerable stress and needed exploring. It seemed she felt neglectful of him, as sex was very important to him prior to the accident. She decided that, as he showed no interest in her sexually, he was not feeling this need. As she felt loving towards her husband but did not feel the need for sexual expression, she decided, after counselling, that they would continue as things now were, but she need not feel guilty about this.

---

Staff often find it difficult to face these issues but it is valuable to address them. Although there may be embarrassment on all sides, there is usually relief that the problem has been noted and considered and does not have to be raised by the patient's partner.

Head injuries often happen to young men at the peak of their sexual activity. As sex fills the mind of most young men it is hardly surprising that young men post head injury, who have much more time on their hands, will think about and may act out sexual feelings and thoughts. This can reach the point of obsession and may need the intervention of a psychologist to develop strategies to cope with this. If inappropriate masturbation is the problem and attempts at changing behaviour have been unsuccessful, distraction techniques can be valuable to occupy the mind and especially the hands.

Disinhibited behaviour can be very distasteful and damages the chance of developing relationships. If the head injury has occurred early in life, for example, immediately before puberty, so that the teenage years are 'lost' in rehabilitation, at a more mature stage there may be a need to try to recapture these lost years and this is not easy.

## Spinal injury problems

As with head injury, the site and severity of the trauma will affect the degree of impairment of function and needs investigating for each individual. Unless there is a coexisting head injury there will be no impairment of awareness of what has happened to the patient. Thus an emotional response to the injury and its effect will not be impaired. Realisation of the extent of the disability will have an effect on self-image, self-esteem and self-confidence. This can influence fears around sustaining current relationships, fear of loss of the relationship and doubts about the ability to attract new partners. Initially, there may be loss of sexual interest and awareness. This can have mixed results, perhaps relief at not needing to sexually perform in response, but also fear that sexual pleasure will never be experienced again, and consequent grief at the loss. Again, a high proportion of patients with spinal injuries are young people where sexual thoughts and fulfilment are high on the agenda. It is important to remember that the time since the injury occurred needs to be taken into consideration. There may be some improvement in the situation over time, often months and perhaps even years. Some couples put their sexual activity 'on hold' and decide to wait and see what the end result may be, but this may mean that no sexual activity occurs in that time and they are denying themselves pleasure meanwhile. They may need reminding that sexual pleasuring involves a whole range of touching and feeling actions of which penetrative sex is only one option.

To perform sexually there are emotional and psychological factors in addition to physical response. Emotional factors will affect desire but also will be affected by other psychological factors such as self-esteem and self-confidence (see Chapter 3). Depending on the site and extent of the injury there may be effects on both sensation and physical response. Loss of sensation will occur below the level of the spinal injury and means that the person is not aware of being touched. Touch is vital in sexual pleasuring. Making love with a light on can be very helpful here as the person can see what is happening and where they are being touched. If they have previous experience of making love, they may be able to rekindle memories from the past, or if not, use their imagination about how the touch may feel. Similarly, a reflexogenic erection can be seen and recalled or fantasised about. Because of the loss of sensation, if a rubber ring is being used to aid or sustain an erection it is essential that one of the partners remembers that it is *in situ* or damage may occur.

Following a spinal injury there will need to be a change in technique of lovemaking. As mobility is impaired in the injured partner the non-injured partner may have to do most of the 'work'. This may mean helping the partner into a suitable position and carrying out movements such as stimulating the penis to obtain an erection, or movement on the penis after penetration. Sometimes involuntary spasms can 'interrupt'. It is important that this does not become an issue and result in avoidance. With a sense of humour, so often essential in coping with disability, the couple can adapt and accept it as a 'nuisance factor'. Spasms can be initiated by the contractions that occur with orgasm. Some people find that their naturally occurring spasms are relieved for hours or days after orgasm.

In general terms, the **higher** the injury to the spine, the better the chances of being able to have erections and ejaculate. Lower back injuries, T12 and below, are more likely to impede the capacity to obtain or sustain an erection if the injury is complete.

If the injury level is T4 or above, one situation to be aware of is that stimulation and excitement, such as induced by orgasm, can result in an exaggerated rise in blood pressure – autonomic dysreflexia. This can also occur with an over-full bladder or bowel or sometimes with procedures such as passing a catheter or having an enema. In women, stimulation of the cervix can have the same result and would be especially likely if inserting an IUD. Anecdotally, it is said that elevation of blood pressure is possible when taking a cervical smear but is very unlikely. All patients and partners should be aware of this potential problem as it has serious import and a risk of cerebral haemorrhage. There is a need to know that it would be experienced as a pounding headache due to a severe rise in blood pressure, together with blotchy skin and blocked nose. If this occurs during lovemaking it is essential to stop immediately and check whether the bladder is the source of the problem. The patient should also sit in an upright position and seek urgent medical advice if the symptoms persist.

The psychological, emotional messages are transmitted via the spinal tract so if it is damaged this transmission is interrupted. It will not be possible to have erections from sexual thoughts, sights or smells. Reflexogenic erections will occur by external stimuli, such as masturbation, or sometimes by being moved (e.g. in a wheelchair over bumpy ground). Internal stimuli such as a full rectum may cause spontaneous erections to occur before, during, or after bowel evacuation. Similarly, stimulation around the rectum may be effective in producing an erection for love making.

All new relationships are an exploration between a couple as to what suits them both. This process continues throughout the relationship. When there has been major trauma, like spinal injury in an ongoing relationship, this new situation also needs exploring. Some previous activities may alter and some are no longer pleasing, or are impossible. It is essential that the couple talk about these thoughts and feelings, otherwise the relationship will suffer. Very frequently these issues do not get discussed. Where physical indication of sexual interest is damaged, verbal communication becomes all the more important. 'Oral sex ' of the verbal variety is even more important in the permanently disabled; sharing what the partners want, or would like to do together, and the feelings that are created.

Where there is limitation or absence of manual stimulation, actual oral sex can be of considerable importance. For some couples this is highly satisfactory but others find it distasteful; as always, it is personal preference and choice that matter. Oral sex does not need to be limited to stimulating the genitalia. Using the mouth and tongue to stimulate other parts of the body can be very effective. There is often an increase in sensitivity above the level of the lesion. This may become so hypersensitive as to reach the level of pain, but often this becomes less acute as time and practice progress.

For women, in addition to the loss of sensation in the genital area and the experience of orgasm being different from before, there may be a decrease in lubrication of the vagina as part of the sexual response. This lack of lubrication can cause difficulties with intercourse. This could mean difficulty in penetration for the partner and although there is loss of sensation, so pain is avoided, there can be trauma to the vaginal walls which may result in an increased tendency to infection. The use of a lubricant to correct this is essential.

# Other neurological conditions

It is impossible to cover all diseases and disabilities in great detail, but general principles apply to all of them:

- what impact has the illness had on the emotional make-up of the individual or the partner?
- what impairment of function has occurred as a result of the disease?
- is the effect permanent or is it a disease of exacerbation and remission?
- is the disease progressive?

Sexual difficulty may be the presenting symptom in some diseases (e.g. multiple sclerosis). It is important to establish a correct diagnosis as sometimes a sexual difficulty is attributed to the disease *per se*. The sexual difficulty may be as a result of the emotional stress of a diagnosis, with all that means to the patient. Careful questioning may elicit that a sexual difficulty may have arisen at other times of severe stress experienced by that person in the distant past.

It has been noted that there is often resolution, or at least improvement, in sexual performance after help has been sought. Obviously, the counselling consultation has not improved the physical capacity to perform (e.g. 'repaired' the nerve damage), but it has benefited the emotional element. Feeling that the problem has been tackled by the patient and that it has been recognised and accepted by the professional will have a beneficial effect. In part this may be a placebo effect but work carried out in a counselling consultation may well have a more lasting outcome.

Where difficulties of communication occur (e.g. in multiple sclerosis or motor neurone disease), the counsellor may have to change their usual method of managing a consultation. Patients may tire easily and be unable to communicate for long before speech becomes jumbled or incoherent. The usual practice of encouraging the patient to talk while the counsellor listens and interprets may need adjusting.

---

**Case study O**

Oliver, who has motor neurone disease, quickly 'ran out of steam' and needed to save his breath and energies to reply and talk in short bursts, then resting to gain the ability to talk some more. The counsellor thus needed to be more proactive and to offer 'guesstimates' for his acceptance or rejection. This change in style can feel quite uncomfortable for the counsellor who is used to a different counselling mode. But in all consultations, effective communication is a basic requirement. Of course, it is essential, as always, to make no assumptions just because communication is difficult.

---

Some patients will not use speech but communicate in other ways (e.g. with Bliss board, Makaton, or by computer). This may mean they will have the ability to communicate with fixed questions or responses or by spelling out what they want to say. The range of fixed questions for them to ask or respond to may not be very applicable to sexuality work. Speech and language service therapists are very adept at developing communication skills and tools and one of the authors (EC) has always found them willing to address the problem of how to communicate in this delicate area.

## Gastrointestinal problems

Fears about bowel control, risk of faecal incontinence due to diarrhoea or anal sphincter failure can inhibit developing sexual relationships and performance. This situation may arise as a result of conditions such as Crohn's disease or ulcerative colitis or after childbirth or surgery. Being governed by a need to be within easy reach of a toilet and worries about whether stimulus will result in 'an accident' is not conducive to a relaxed sex life. Even after repair for anal incontinence, it will take some time to gain confidence in control. These concerns and anxieties may lead to avoidance of sexual activity and strain the relationship. The partner may also have anxieties.

If manual evacuation is necessary for bowel management (e.g. as with spinal injury), it is helpful to have the bowel cleared before lovemaking. Evacuation sometime previously (i.e. not immediately before) separates these practicalities from the lovemaking. This procedure may be performed by the partner in their role of carer. As mentioned elsewhere, this may cause conflict in the lover/nurse-carer role and so may best be carried out by a health professional (e.g. district nurse).

For some patients, management of the disease or disability may require bowel surgery and the formation of a temporary or permanent stoma. Much valuable work can be done in addressing both the emotional and practical worries of both the patient and their partner as to how this could, or will, affect their relationship or sexual performance, prior to the surgery being performed. If the patient is in a relationship they may prefer to attend alone or with their partner. Similarly, the partner may like to be able to express their worries alone or with the patient present. There are advantages and disadvantages in all these combinations. Shared consultations mean both partners are aware of the same information, but either or both may feel inhibited in expressing their anxieties in front of the other partner for fear of causing them distress. Fears may concern sequelae from surgery, such as inevitable nerve damage, which may result in a permanent effect on sexual performance (e.g. inability to obtain erections or to ejaculate). These need to be discussed with the surgeon, and practical solutions considered (see Chapter 4).

Following major surgery, many patients experience temporary impairment of performance or desire and need a period of recuperation. However, there may well be an improvement in physical performance with time.

There may be anxieties about the effect that a stoma's appearance will have on the partner. Will they be distressed or disgusted? Will the partner no longer find them attractive? This may be a reflection of how the patients feel about themselves (i.e. that they are distressed or disgusted or see themselves as undesirable). There will be a particular concern about the partner's reaction at first sight. In forming new relationships there may be anxieties about how to tell the new, or prospective, partner about the stoma. When clothed, the stoma is invisible but in intimate situations it is difficult to conceal. Some people feel very self-conscious about the stoma and feel as if the fact they have one is branded across their forehead. Initially, some women find the wearing of a garment such as a teddy* helpful, as it can be both alluring and concealing. It is more difficult for men but sometimes boxer shorts can be helpful or adaptable. With confidence, nudity becomes less of a problem.

There can be many anxieties about the bag, especially whether it will leak, make a noise, smell, or come off. Some people find it helpful to use a cover for their bag. It is wise for the patient and/or the partner to address these issues with the stoma care nurse, who will have experience in discussing these matters. These fears are often far worse in prospect than in actuality. It is important that they are faced, or wariness and anxiety may result in sexual difficulty which could have been avoided.

Attention to the diet to avoid particularly eruptive evacuations of the stoma, or wind, may be necessary. It is good practice to ensure that the bag is empty prior to lovemaking (if there is time). A relaxed attitude helps avoid accidents and coping with them if they occur.

Both the patient and the partner may feel that physical damage may be caused by sexual activity, particularly penetration. Explicit discussion may be needed concerning the anatomical relationship of the urogenital and bowel systems. Initially, gentleness – as confidence is gained – is an advantage in lovemaking.

## Other disabilities affecting body image

Any disability or illness that alters a person's appearance has the potential to affect that person's self-confidence and self-esteem. This may alter their ability to form relationships, and emotional factors may then impair performance, although the physical prerequisites for sexual activity are intact. The opportunity to express these feelings can be very helpful and ongoing counselling can be offered.

Where the disability results in functional loss (e.g. loss of a limb), there will be both emotional and practical aspects. Even though the genitalia and necessary vascular and neurological systems are intact, the practicalities of sexual performance may

*Teddy: a short petticoat reaching to the top of the thighs.

need addressing. For instance, the loss of a hand or arm will need a change in technique, for stimulation of the partner, or for self-stimulation. The loss of a leg, or legs, may make some positions for intercourse difficult or impossible (see Chapter 4 on positions)

## The reproductive system

Disease, disability or trauma affecting the sexual organs can have a marked affect on sexuality. Obviously, where there is a change to the external appearance there may be effects on body image with emotional consequences. Loss of, or damage to, the penis, testicles, scrotum, vagina or labia will often cause grief, which needs to be expressed. In addition, there may be interference with function. This may result in many anxieties in addition to practical difficulties. For women, damage to or loss of the breast can affect their confidence, the breast being so much a part of a woman's appearance and sexuality. As with the patient with a stoma, being naked is a vulnerable experience, especially in the early days, or when entering new relationships.

For those women where the internal organs, uterus and ovaries or even just the cervix following an abnormal smear, have been surgically 'assaulted', there may also be emotional difficulties to overcome. **Pre**-operative or **pre**-treatment counselling is valuable. The woman needs to be able to work through and express her feelings as to how this impinges on her sexuality, especially if fertility is affected. Some women seem unable to deal with this until later, when the acute phase is over. Learning to live without genital organs may cause both physical and emotional problems. Some men and women can feel very third-rate and less of a man or woman than their peers. For some people, the knowledge that they will be unable to have children is very distressing and this may affect the image they have of themselves. Even those people who were adamant that they would not have children feel grief and anger at their loss of choice. These factors may affect forming relationships or sexual performance. Counselling is very important in this context. Hormone replacement therapy (HRT) should always be offered to counteract the hormone-deficiency effect of bilateral oophorectomy or bilateral orchidectomy.

Young people who have had chemotherapy for malignant disease early in their lives often have concerns which need exploring about the effects of the treatment on their sexuality and fertility.

## Terminal illness

For many people, professionals and non-professionals, putting the words 'sexuality' and 'dying' together is a challenging concept. It is more difficult than the concept of 'sexuality and disability'. This makes the aspect of need, or problems, difficult to raise for both the patient and their partner and/or the professional. Of course, there are many other issues to address at this time and for some couples sex is low on the agenda, but for others where it has been a significant part of their lives it is sad if this area is overlooked. As always there will be integration of emotional and physical factors and these need addressing and exploring. The time of diagnosis, or setbacks in progress of the condition, will have an emotional impact on all aspects of the couple's lives. Some will find solace in the closeness of physical contact but for others it will interfere with their expression of sexual needs. There may be fear in the partner of making demands on the patient who is already very unwell. In the past, partners have expressed anxiety that they may 'catch' the disease but this seems less prevalent now – this was particularly true in the case of genital organ malignancy. Where such irrational fear exists it is a powerful barrier to sexual activity.

After counselling, there may be some improvement in the ability to perform as emotional aspects have been explored, but as the disease progresses physical factors arise such as fatigue and debility. The closeness of physical contact and simply touching may be comforting to both and, as always, communication – putting feelings into words – is important and needs to be encouraged.

---

**Case study P**

Patrick was diagnosed with a malignant disease that was progressive. He was dismayed to find that he was experiencing difficulty in obtaining and sustaining an erection. The sexual content of his relationship with his wife had always been very important. They were concerned at this loss and wondered whether it was permanent and if so what could be done. Exploring the situation with them, their feelings about this difficulty were discussed at length. How much of the difficulty to perform was due to emotion and how much was due to his physical condition was not clear. Practical options (see Chapter 4) were explored. Patrick's performance improved and they were both very pleased with this. Some months later he was in contact again, because the problem recurred as his physical condition deteriorated. He opted to use intracavernosal injections. These proved very successful and he was able to use these for the last few months of his life. He and his wife felt that they were able to continue to enjoy their last months together in a way that suited them. It is important to address these situations as a matter of urgency. When Patrick was referred for the injection he was initially placed on a waiting list. But this is totally unacceptable when time is limited.

## Hospitalisation

When people are hospitalised long term (e.g. in rehabilitation units), the unit becomes their home. However, it lacks the privacy enjoyed at home and some couples find this inhibitory. As couples have said, 'it is not that we want to do anything but we lose the opportunity for intimate moments or conversations'. Staff sometimes say they need to be able to enter a room at any time for safety reasons. However, if a couple are together, one of the couple would usually be able to summon help in an emergency. Simple measures such as 'do not disturb' notices, which can be displayed on the door as in hotels, can be very helpful and much appreciated by the couple.

## Conditions that may result in disability

### Diabetes

Although many people with diabetes are able to live their lives without impairment by keeping their diabetes under control, for others the complications of diabetes may lead to disability. As with all disability there will be both an emotional and physical reaction. If diabetes has been diagnosed in childhood there may be issues about feeling different, set apart, which inhibit self-confidence. Diagnosis later in life may be accepted or seen as a major problem and evidence of physical decline. Physical complications of diabetes may include neurological and vascular damage. Diabetic retinopathy can result in visual impairment, with obvious results. For men the most striking effect may be on their capacity to have or to sustain erections. Erectile dysfunction may be the presenting symptom in diabetes and all men complaining of erectile dysfunction should be checked for glycosuria. At an earlier stage if diabetes is poorly controlled erectile problems may be improved by improving the level of control. When neurological damage has occurred it is irreversible (but now treatable by intracavernosal injections or sildenafil). Vascular damage may result in ischaemia, gangrene and loss of a limb, usually the leg. This can have a profound effect on sexual performance due to damage to body image and self-esteem, in addition to some practical problems (see case study D). Women whose sexual function is less severely impaired than men can find lack of lubrication in the vagina and recurrent candidiasis to be a problem. These can, of course, be treated by lubricants for dryness and antifungals for the candida. It has been known for hypoglycaemia to occur if lovemaking is prolonged and vigorous. This is offputting but can be avoided by appropriate food or drink. One couple found a tray of coffee and crackers by the bed helpful!

## Epilepsy

If epilepsy is well controlled so that there are no, or only occasional, seizures the likelihood of disabling complications is minimal. There may, however, be psychological effects as a response to the diagnosis and its repercussions. These are mainly sociological, with restrictions of employment and some sporting activity. Loss of the driving licence after seizures may be a major blow. If the onset of seizures is late there may be anger and grief at the restrictions. These losses affect how the people perceive themselves or feel they may be perceived by others. Self-esteem may well be affected. The emotional response to diminished self-worth can then affect sexual desire and performance.

Epilepsy can be associated with a physical or learning disability (e.g. cerebral palsy). Young people who were diagnosed in childhood may feel different and set apart as do those diagnosed with diabetes in childhood. This may inhibit confidence. Unfortunately, even in the 1990s some people attach a stigma to being epileptic.

If the seizures are poorly controlled, especially if there is status epilepticus, there may be long-term physical consequences such as hemiparesis with its attendant effects on body image. In some women, seizures occur more frequently premenstrually. One young woman had status epilepticus in the three days preceding her period on a regular basis. This was cause for concern. Consideration was given to eliminating the menstrual cycle in an endeavour to prevent this condition. Because of the possible increased risk of cerebral thrombosis, Depo-Provera was prescribed rather than combined oral contraception. This proved very effective in abolishing the cycle and the seizures.

As mentioned in Chapter 6, there may be drug interaction between anticonvulsants and contraceptive hormones and adjustment needs to be made. Practitioners fitting intrauterine devices (IUDs) need to be aware of the possibility of a seizure occurring during the insertion and prepare accordingly.

Some anticonvulsant drugs have a sedating effect and this may reduce libido. Some people who have epilepsy or their partners are anxious that the excitement of sexual activity and orgasm may induce a seizure. Fortunately, this is reported as occurring only rarely.[1] Anxiety about this can have an inhibitory effect on becoming involved in sexual activity. In addition, there are concerns that the drugs taken to prevent seizures may affect the fetus, and pre-conception counselling is vital (see Chapter 5).

# Reference

1. Bancroft J (1989) Sexual aspects of medical practice. In: J Bancroft (ed) *Human Sexuality and Its Problems.* Churchill Livingstone, Edinburgh.

# Further reading

Anon (1990) *Life Style: you and your ostomy. No 4: Love and Sex.* Hollister, Reading.

Coughlan AK and Morgan MR (1995) *Personal and Sexual Relationships Following Head Injury.* Headway/National Head Injuries Association, Nottingham.

Mooney TO, Cole TM and Chilgren RA (1975) *Sexual Options for Paraplegics and Quadriplegics.* Little, Brown and Company, Boston MA.

Spinal Injuries Association (1993) *Sexuality and Spinal Cord Injury: heterosexual men.* SIA, London.

Spinal Injuries Association (1993) *Sexuality and Spinal Cord Injury: gay men.* SIA, London.

Spinal Injuries Association (1993) *Sexuality and Spinal Cord Injury: lesbian women.* SIA, London.

Spinal Injuries Association (1993) *Sexuality and Spinal Cord Injury: heterosexual women.* SIA, London.

SPOD leaflets.

# CHAPTER 9

# A further look at learning disability

## Screening

An important area of healthcare often overlooked in people with learning disability is screening and raising awareness of the fact that such problems as breast or testicular lumps can occur. It seems to be a myth that if people have one health problem, such as a disability, then they will not develop the same health problems that the rest of the population experience. In part this is another aspect of the non-acceptance of people with disabilities as being sexual individuals. When the person has a learning disability and impairment of understanding there is a general reluctance to raise the problem of physically checking the body, especially the more intimate parts such as breasts and testicles.

It is important that parents or professional carers who are involved with body care are aware what to look for (e.g. changes in appearance of the breast or testicular swelling) so that these can be reported. There is a hesitancy to carry out 'hands on' checking as this can be misinterpreted. It is possible for health professionals to explain these procedures to the carer or to the person with the disability in the presence of the carer if consent is given. The carer can then encourage the person to look at their breasts or to examine their testicles (at an appropriate frequency). In support of this, leaflets are helpful, especially those of a pictorial nature. In Southampton, the learning disability team has produced a illustrated leaflet on testicular examination for people with learning disability. Exploring this issue with the local oncologist has raised support, as he reports that these men referred with testicular cancer usually attend for their first consultation when the tumour is at an advanced stage, which reduces the very good outcome that can be expected from attending at an early stage. It is hoped that this leaflet will be circulated widely to men with learning disability, and their carers, to raise awareness of this important health check – but **without** creating undue anxiety.

Concerns about any misinterpretation of examination by carers need to be addressed and written into care plans to give protection to both staff and clients in this vulnerable area. Many mothers caring for their daughters have continued to bathe them and are willing to monitor their daughter's breasts.

In Britain, women are routinely called for breast screening from the age of 50 to 64 years and for cervical screening from the age of 20 to 64 years, provided they are registered with a general practitioner. So women with disabilities should also receive their notifications. However, it has been known for general practitioners, or others, to make a decision that this is not going to be necessary due to the person's learning disability and the woman not informed. Although there may be reasons why the woman does not need cervical screening (e.g. the cervix has been surgically removed as part of hysterectomy), the need for breast screening remains for all women.

## Breast screening

It would obviously be confusing, and possibly frightening, for a woman to attend unprepared for breast screening. A clear explanation of the procedure needs to be made within the level of the woman's understanding. Most women find a mammogram uncomfortable. For some with severe or profound learning disability, examination may be impossible but it should never be dismissed out of hand. The situation needs exploring on an individual basis.

# Cervical screening

This type of screening can be more difficult due to its intrusive nature. Again, decisions may be taken by health professionals or carers not to screen, but the situation needs individual investigation. For each woman, an assessment needs to be made of the benefit and need for screening and the stress and sometimes fear that is likely to be experienced by that particular woman. A careful sexual history is important in this context. The woman may well be able to give information as to whether she has ever been sexually active. Such a woman will be in a position to understand explanations and to make an informed choice, provided the explanation is given in a way that is intelligible to her. She will then be in a position to consent.

If the woman is unclear about this herself, she may be known, by health professionals or carers, to have been sexually active. As sexual intercourse can be a risk factor for cervical disease this knowledge is important in assessing what risks there may be for that woman. If the woman has never had penetrative vaginal sex then the likelihood of abnormal findings is greatly reduced and the distress caused by the examination outweighs the benefits.

Conversely, if the woman has been sexually very active, perhaps with many partners, then screening becomes essential, and, of course, if women have symptoms, such as vaginal bleeding, an examination is essential. Examination then needs to be carried out, as part of an examination under anaesthesia, if necessary, but this is a clinical investigation and not screening. It needs to be remembered that women who have been sexually abused involving sexual intercourse many years previously still need screening, even if they are not currently sexually active.

The person who is to take the smear, doctor or nurse, may have some anxieties about carrying out the examination. There will be concerns around consent and the person taking the cervical smear can have worries about the interpretation the patient will make about the procedure. The practitioner may feel that they are being intrusive and abusive, as if they are carrying out an assault. It is important that these feelings are explored, but do not cloud judgement when assessing whether the smear is necessary or not. The key to reducing these anxieties is communication and explanation to the patient. Often, forward planning is very valuable here with work being done, with the woman, about her body and examinations. Pictures may be very useful in this context. Sometimes the person likely to take the smear needs to be involved in this forward planning. It can be time consuming but worthwhile.

---

**Case study Q**

Queenie is very frightened of doctors and is phobic that all doctors use needles. She has been in an institution most of her life and has been examined there. She now lives in the community. She is known to have been very sexually active over the years so a cervical smear is advisable. The community nurse has worked hard with Queenie on the need for general health checks, starting with the least sensitive aspect, such as eyes and feet, and visiting the dentist. Queenie came to the clinic but was too frightened to enter the building. It was therefore necessary for the doctor to visit her at home so that they could get to know each other. This consultation focused on the areas Queenie had worked through before, but then went on to talking about abdominal and internal examinations. During the consultation Queenie offered to come to the clinic with the nurse. In due course it is hoped that Queenie will eventually agree to an examination. The doctor was able to accommodate this problem within her work in the learning disability team, but it could well be too great an investment of time for a busy general practitioner.

---

If the decision is made, on balance, not to carry out a cervical smear then those involved with the woman should be aware that symptoms, such as abnormal bleeding, should always be reported so that they can be investigated.

Health professionals, especially community nurses, are often involved in organising women's or men's groups. At these groups it is an ideal opportunity to highlight and explore these health issues in a safe environment.

## The menopause

A milestone health event that occurs in all women is the climacteric, or menopause. Over the years there has been a myth that people with learning disabilities are 'forever young'. This is probably because of their unsophisticated behaviour and the myth that they are forever in a child-like state and do not develop sexually. As it is necessary to be aware that hormonal changes affect all young people, male and female, at adolescence, it is also necessary to be aware that changes also occur at the menopause. There may be mood swings and in women with severe or profound learning disability these mood swings may result in exacerbation of behavioural problems. It can be very confusing for the woman to feel these changes without any understanding of why. It may be noticed that the woman has other physical symptoms, such as flushes and sweats, or difficulties with the urinary tract such as an increase in night rising to pass urine. If dysuria, urethral irritation and vaginal dryness occur during the menopause this may result in an increase in rubbing or touching the genitals and this can increase discomfort and occur at inappropriate times and places.

In addition to monitoring for menopausal symptoms and consideration of treatment, possibly with hormone replacement therapy (HRT), the 'hidden' benefits of the latter in prevention of osteoporosis and cardiovascular disease need also to be taken into account. If it is decided that HRT should be used there may be problems regarding the route of administration. Compliance and the ability to swallow oral formulations may not be possible and the patch formulation needs to be discussed. Some patients find picking at, and removing, the patch irresistible. Unless there has been a hysterectomy, current practice suggests that the use of oestrogen gels alone is unsuitable and the addition of progestogens necessary. Currently, studies are underway in Southampton and London concerning progestogen creams. However, many women have already been using these creams for menopausal symptoms but until now there has been no clinical assessment of how effective they are in the prevention of osteoporosis.

## Inappropriate behaviour

The reason for referral is not uncommonly that a person with a learning disability is behaving inappropriately. It is important not to take this at face value but to make careful enquiry as to what the behaviour is. The client is not usually the complainant, so the assessment of inappropriate behaviour is made by others, family, carers, the public, other professionals. What we each consider to be inappropriate is very subjective and depends on upbringing, and other social and moral beliefs. Objectively, the behaviour may not in itself be inappropriate but the circumstances may be inappropriate (e.g. masturbating in the supermarket or at the dinner table is inappropriate). Care is needed in separating this antisocial behaviour from the activity itself, so that it is not labelled inappropriate with connotations that may go with that such as 'dirtiness'. As previously stressed, unless the person with the learning disability has been given certain boundaries, about what is and is not inappropriate behaviour, how are they going to know?

The situation may be a result of individual action, such as masturbating inappropriately, or may involve inappropriate behaviour towards other people. Unless some guidance is given people will tend to act as they feel, like eating when hungry. Sexual feelings or interest may be indulged as they arise.

Most young men, with or without a disability, are sexually aware and take notice of women or men according to their orientation. Many men will have sexual thoughts and fantasies and may become sexually aroused. However, most people without learning disability are aware that society has 'rules' of acceptable and unacceptable behaviour. People with a learning disability may not be aware of these rules and behave as they feel, talking to strangers in an unsuitable way, perhaps being sexually explicit or by inappropriate touching. Often, the young man has no insight into the consequences of this behaviour either in regard to how the recipient will feel or consequences for themselves (e.g. allegations of assault).

It is important that both men and women with a learning disability are taught that they and their bodies need respect and should not be taken advantage of. Sexual contact should always be with mutual, two-way consent, explicit or maybe implicit (which is more difficult to establish/prove).

People with learning disabilities often find it difficult to communicate their point of view. This may be because they feel they must comply with whatever they are told to do, but is sometimes due to fear of the consequences of non-compliance. This makes the person, man or woman, open to exploitation and sometimes sexual abuse. It is not uncommon for women, especially younger women, to feel unable to say 'no' even if they wish to do so. Sometimes they will be able to say 'no' but in such an ineffectual way that they are ignored.

---

**Case study R**

Rose is a young woman with a learning disability who is often taken advantage of. She often feels obliged to comply with a man's sexual demands. She is unable to see potential problems ahead and will put herself in risky positions (e.g. go in a car with someone whom she knows little or distrusts). If she asks anyone for assistance in coping with her everyday life she has become accustomed to that person wanting sexual favours as payment. Conversely, she sees if she is amenable to their demands, they may be more willing to help her. At first, Rose could not see that there was any choice. She accepted that she should do as she is told. She had no insight to her own worth and rights over her body. Over time, she is beginning to be more aware and assertive. She will now say 'no' and has taken action against those who ignore it. With continued help, it is hoped that more notice will be taken of her wishes.

---

It can be very helpful to have input from the learning disability team to manage these situations better. Joint working with community nurses and psychologists can be effective here.

## Response to sexual behaviour

Witnessing inappropriate behaviour or behaviour that is perceived as inappropriate can cause alarm in the bystander be they relative, carer, professional or member of the public. As stated earlier, the judgement of appropriate/inappropriate behaviour can vary. Alarm can be caused by any evidence of sexual awareness, as there is a fear that it will escalate and that there will be consequences for the person involved, the person they are relating to, and sometimes the carer who feels they will be held responsible. This can result in overreaction which may be punitive. This may be by segregating the sexes, a 'locking up your daughters' type of response, to avoid risk. Although this may be effective it denies that person or couple the opportunity to enjoy relationships which may or may not be sexual – the denial of normal human interaction. It is important, of course, to ensure that relationships are freely entered into and that the couple are as well informed as possible to minimise risks, both emotional and physical. A low-key response enables the situation to be explored and discussed with the person/couple, and safeguards to be made without the negative feelings of doing something 'wrong' and being blamed, which the person with learning disability often experiences.

Sometimes, ongoing relationships develop which are valuable and pleasurable to both partners and they may have hopes to marry or live together and plan accordingly.

---

**Case studies S and T**

Samantha and Trevor are both in their thirties and are in love. They enjoy being together. This has, at times, caused problems at the day centre as they like to kiss and cuddle in public, which is inappropriate. Work needed to be done with them around this point and to explore what they understood about relationships, including the responsibilities involved, as well as ensuring that they were well informed of the consequences of expressing their sexual interest in each other. As is often the case, sex education had either not been given or was not recognised as being relevant at the time.

---

It is important, of course, when counselling couples to be non-judgemental and not to apply values or codes of behaviour upon them from the counsellor's viewpoint. Couples with learning disabilities, as others without a disability, will need to decide for themselves what is right and wrong within a caring relationship. Being more susceptible to doing as they are told, people with learning disability may find that they cannot test the boundaries and accept the behaviour that the parent or carers feel they should. This can cause problems, for example, when a couple who are encouraged to become engaged as a sign of commitment, and intend to marry, are told they must abide by the code of no sex except kissing and cuddling until they do marry, which they and many others feel to be the correct way to live. However, they are often not seen to be able to marry due to their learning disabilities but are led to believe that they will. This is an uncomfortable double standard.

## Masturbation

Masturbation is normal sexual behaviour for both boys and girls, men and women. However, as mentioned in Chapter 7 it is not uncommonly carried out at an inappropriate time or in an inappropriate place. It is important in dealing with this behaviour not to be punitive and 'slap wrist' about it. It is easy to give out very negative messages by reacting sharply in giving the impression that this is the behaviour of 'dirty old men'. Exploring the need to masturbate, accepting that and encouraging appropriate expression by laying down boundaries as to when and where in a low-key, matter of fact way can be helpful. There may be a need to repeat and reinforce these boundaries on a recurring basis until this pattern of behaviour becomes accepted. There is usually more anxiety about masturbation being performed by young men because it is more obvious both in the activity and in the result. Women may be more discreet in some ways in that they may rock upon their heel as a means of stimulating themselves. This is not so obvious, however it can be more obvious for instance, where the clothes are raised and the hand thrust into the pants to stimulate, perhaps in public.

## Further reading

Craft A (ed) (1994) *Practice Issues in Sexuality and Learning Disabilities*. Routledge, London.
Craft A (1987) *Mental Handicap and Sexuality: issues and perspectives*. Costello, Tunbridge Wells.

# Postscript

Health professionals and social workers are well placed to address many of the issues raised in relation to sexuality and disability. By recognising, accepting and valuing the need of people with disability to express their sexuality, as is their right and the right of all individuals, difficulties can be addressed and overcome to enable them to have the choice of sexual expression – like everyone else. People with disabilities are people first and not a breed apart.

# Additional Reading

Brearley G and Birchley P (1994) *Counselling in Disability and Illness* (2nd edition). Mosby, London.

Campion MJ (1995) *Who's Fit to be a Parent?* Routledge, London.

Carson D (ed) (1987) *The Law and the Sexuality of People with Mental Handicaps.* University of Southampton Law Faculty, Southampton.

Gunn MJ (1991) *Sex and the Law: a brief guide for staff working with people with learning difficulties* (3rd edition). Family Planning Association, London.

Keith L (ed) (1994) *Mustn't Grumble: writings by disabled women.* Women's Press, London.

Lincoln R (ed) (1992) *Psychosexual Medicine: a study of underlying themes.* Chapman and Hall, London.

McK.Norrie K (1991) *Family Planning Practice and the Law.* Dartmouth, Aldershot.

McPherson A and Waller D (eds) (1997) *Women's Problems in General Practice.* Oxford University Press, Oxford.

Montford H and Skrine R (eds) (1993) *Contraceptive Care: meeting individuals' needs.* Chapman and Hall, London.

Morris J (1996) *Pride Against Prejudice: transforming attitudes to disability* (3rd edition). Women's Press, London.

Skrine R (1997) *Blocks and Freedoms in Sexual Life: a handbook of psychosexual medicine.* Radcliffe Medical Press, Oxford.

# Index